An Introspective Journey

An Introspective Journey
Copyright © 2018
Paula Sarver

Cover concept and design by Jonathan Grisham.

All rights reserved. No part of this book may be reproduced, stored in a retrieval system, or transmitted in any form or by any means—electronic, mechanical, photocopy, recording or otherwise—without the prior written permission of the publisher. The only exception is brief quotations for review purposes.

Published by WordCrafts Press
Cody, Wyoming 82414
www.wordcrafts.net

An Introspective Journey

A Memoir of
Living with Alzheimer's

Paula Sarver

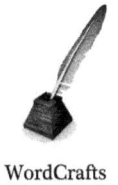

WordCrafts

Contents

GETTING TO KNOW MY FAMILY 1
LIFE GROWING UP 6
CAREGIVING 17
THE EARLY YEARS OF ALZHEIMER'S 26
MOUNTING LIMITATIONS 49
NO MORE HIDING FROM REALITY 74
SOMETHING'S WRONG; PEOPLE NOTICE 105
GETTING HELP 145
A NEW WAY OF LIFE 160
NEVER GIVE UP 163
FROM THE ALZHEIMER'S ASSOCIATION 171
ABOUT THE AUTHOR 172

Chapter 1

GETTING TO KNOW MY FAMILY

"Come on troop," called out Mom and Dad as we set out on a trip. With 4 kids our vacations were mostly limited to visiting family. We piled into the old station wagon with all the seats laying down as the four of us sat in a circle playing endless games until we made it to our destination, Christmas at Grandmother and Granddaddy's house.

The whole family was there, aunts, uncles, and cousins. Walking into the house we smelled the gumbo that had been cooking all day. The aroma would lead us straight to the kitchen to sneak a peek or perhaps get a taste. My Aunt Shelly smacked all of us with a bright red kiss on our cheek as we came in. Cousins, Andrea and Neal, ran to greet us as we went to the backyard to play making sure never to step on Grandmother's monkey grass planted on the edge of the yard. The meal was topped off with an incredibly tasty cake that had fallen apart during the baking. I sat at the counter watching Grandmother prepare everything for our family. She apologized for the cake not looking pretty.

"That's OK," I told her. "The uglier it is, the better it tastes and that's what matters."

Grandmother was prim and proper. Everything had its place

and her house was always immaculate. She was modest and timid, the perfect lady with such discipline in her actions and her emotions. Her posture was exact when sitting up or standing, almost rigid. Never have I seen her slouch or merely rest her shoulders. Even when she drove, her hands were firmly placed at 10 and 2 on the steering wheel. Like clockwork, she ate at the same time, got up in the morning and went to bed at the same time.

I have no memory of her being in good health, playing or running around, even with her grandkids. Her idea of playing with her grandchildren was playing checkers or cards at a table. Even when the family got together and went out in the evening, she never came along but would stay at home. We just accepted her as she was, frail and weak. She always took a ton of medicine. I even played "grandmother" when I'd take a gum wrapper and placed pretend powder in it to take for a headache. That was her ritual, several times a day to take an aspirin powder to ease her pain.

After an incredible dinner the dishes were immediately cleaned up. The adults would sit around the living room visiting. Us girls, Maria, Paula, and Andrea usually played with our dolls while the boys, Jude, Chris, and Neal would play with cars. Time came for opening presents. Everyone was given something of equal value. Grandmother and Granddaddy were sticklers in making sure everything was even among their children and grandchildren. Even on our birthdays, we knew to expect a $13 check. Why $13? I never knew except perhaps they remained on a budget and when they divided the money out, that was everyone's share.

By now it was late afternoon and time to visit "Old Grandma," my granddad's mother. She lived in an old wooden home. Her demeanor was just kind and sweet as a great grandmother should be. She always had cookies or hard candies to offer us. As time went on Mom realized she was using her food stamps to buy

Getting to Know my Family

treats for us when we came. She sacrificed something for herself to have something to offer us. After that time, we no longer told her when we were coming, but surprised her so she would not feel obligated to buy us something.

We enjoyed going to her meager home. It's difficult to explain why. Perhaps it is because of the love we felt walking through the door. The house in south Louisiana was not air-conditioned. There was no TV to watch or toys to play with. Old Grandma only spoke French, so all the adults in the room visited speaking a language foreign to me.

And there was Clenis, her grown mentally handicapped child. Clenis could not talk. He sat in a rocking chair most of the day. Clenis always had a pack of Juicy Fruit gum in his pocket. He'd walk up to each of us and stick a piece of gum in our faces, grunting. If we did not accept his offer, he'd get angry and persist. We quickly learned never to refuse his gum offer.

Atile Vidrine, Old Grandma, was Mom's role model and inspiration since she exhibited the greatest love Mom had ever experienced as she was growing up. I was also drawn to this incredible lady and wanted to know her more and be able to communicate with her. She was the reason, when I entered high school, I took French as my foreign language. I remember the day we went to Old Grandma's house and Mom told her I was taking French in school so we could start talking. She was so happy.

To say her life was hard would be grossly understated. As a child her father died, and her mother remarried. Her mother's new husband did not want children, so her mother sent Atile to another family member to raise her. She moved to different families where she worked for her stay. Mom told me a story about how she had even run away at one time to escape this life she had been thrown into.

She married young and her first-born was born with severe mental disabilities. Due to the severity of his disabilities, the state wanted to put him away in a home, but she refused to give up her child. She also had four other children, my granddad, Remie, LeRoy, Jim, and her only daughter, Rose.

Her husband died at an early age and she was left caring for their children. In addition to that, she cared for her mother-in-law who was "senile." The combination of caring for her mother-in-law while raising her children with a handicapped child who could not talk or understand was toxic. Her mother-in-law spoke out of her head and did "crazy" things. Atile had no choice but to keep her mother-in-law locked in a room for her safety and keep her disabled son, Clenis, away from her.

I never did meet this lady because she passed before I was born, but as Mom talked about her, we are certain, she also suffered from Alzheimer's Disease. In 1982, Atile went into a coma and remained that way for two years before she passed away in 1984. I questioned God as to why he would leave someone in that state for so long. The strain on the family was great. Mom, in her wisdom, was convinced that it was God's grace for Clenis. He had only been cared for by his mother and would not have comprehended this sudden loss. During her coma, he was allowed to sit by her side as he discovered she could not help him. He learned to rely on others and let others help him. I learned much about God's mercy from this experience and how God loves all of his children.

Clenis lived four more years and died in 1988 at the age of 74.

As the years past, the disease infiltrated more family members. When Granddad was in the nursing home, mom flew with him to his brother Jim's funeral. Jim died in a hospital, covered with bed sores. He had become bedridden. His Alzheimer's had gotten to the point that he'd express a pain, but when asked where he couldn't tell the staff where the pain was because he'd forgotten.

Granddad's sister, Rose, was much younger than Remie. She was more like a close cousin to Mom than an aunt. Rose embodied the character of her mother. She always had a kind word and a smile to offer. Her love for life and everyone was overflowing and contagious. Graciousness, compassion, and generosity were evident, especially during the years that she cared for her mother, Atile. She also was tormented with Alzheimer's Disease later in her life.

Mom and Dad went to visit her one day after she had been placed in a home. Tears fell down Mom's face as she recalled her visit. Rose's face was now blank almost all of the time. Mom looked through the door of her room as Rose rested. She was curled up in the fetal position. It was almost more than Mom could bear watching what this disease had done to someone she loved so much. In 2014, at the age of 84, Rose's life here on Earth came to an end. She is no longer prisoned in this world with a mind that can't remember or express herself.

My first knowledge of this disease came from the announcement of my grandmother's sister, Rita, being diagnosed. We were all shocked, especially my grandmother. Grandmother would visit Rita and say how sad it was, watching what this disease was doing to her. Little did she know it would not be long before the same diagnosis would come to her. Another of Grandmother's brothers, Ambrose, was found one evening sleeping in a ditch as he left his house and wandered around unsure of where to go.

Mom was haunted by the thought that one day she may also be under the spell of Alzheimer's that takes away the ability to act and react appropriately.

Chapter 2

LIFE GROWING UP

We were a traditional American family with mom staying at home with the kids and dad working several jobs to make ends meet. His work was mostly hard labor at plants, driving trucks as a delivery man, repairing appliances, and then in the oilfield. Mom was supported and strengthened through the years by her faith in Jesus Christ. Her faith was solidified through the example of her grandmother, Atile. It was her personal relationship with Jesus that held her together to manage the family.

Neither Mom or Dad had a college education. Mom and Dad, Paul and Beverly, were married in Dec. of 1965, soon after Dad returned from his service in the US Air Force. Nine months later came their first-born, Maria, in September 1966. I was next in January of 1968 with two more children Jude, in April 1969 and Chris, in May 1970. After this, the priest gave them permission to use contraceptives which stopped the flow of children every year.

Mom bore the load of raising four young children on her own with dad working most of the time. Our lives were structured with set times in getting up, eating meals, and going to bed. Church played an integral part of our lives. Christ-like behaviors were modeled by both Mom and Dad. We were deeply loved and were shown compassion and tenderness with a good dose of discipline when needed. Standards and expectations were high. Everyone was treated with respect. Mom's hands were full in caregiving and did little for herself. Through the years her hobbies kept her busy painting, drawing, ceramics, cross stitching, cake decorating, and interior design.

Once we were all in school, Mom joined the workforce to help pay the bills. We lived a simple life, but had lots of laughter and joy in our home. We entertained ourselves through home-made plays, songs, and writing poetry. It was not unusual to walk into the living room or a bedroom that was filled with sheets being used as our tents or see us play in the backyard climbing trees and in our homemade cardboard clubhouses. Refrigerator boxes that dad brought home were a treasure. God always provided for us. We often wore hand-me-downs and Mom sewed lots of dresses for us girls which we proudly wore.

As a child, I didn't think about anyone much but me. Now, as an adult, I marvel at the way we were raised with such love knowing the sacrifices that my parents must have made through the years. The craziness of four children so young and close in age must have worn out Mom and Dad. Not to mention the worry I know we put them through when we came home after curfew and other poor choices we made when we were teens. What I didn't realize was how they were able to be so calm and deal with the four of us and keep their marriage and their love strong through the years. I've discovered their strength came from above. Their unshakable faith held them together and held them strong.

I was a strong-willed child with a mind of my own. I didn't like people to tell me what to do and when I was told something, it required an explanation. I functioned much the same way when I wanted my way. Mom and Dad always listened. I would think everything out and had an answer for all perceived questions ahead of time. I stated my case rationally and usually got my way.

This is where my faith story begins. I saw first-hand what Christianity looked like in my parents, but I didn't understand everything that was said and done in the church setting. I must have driven Mom crazy with questions about Christ. She never told me I was wrong with any of my thoughts but directed me to answers. I was allowed to explore and learn about Christ on my own. I was given the freedom to experience Christ personally in my way, in my time.

I recall a conversation with mom one day while she was putting on her make-up. With four kids, there wasn't much time to sit and talk quietly. I kept asking her questions about her faith. I wanted to know how she could know without a shadow of doubt, when there wasn't anything tangible I could see. I remember her putting down her make-up brush and taking my hands in hers. She looked at me directly in my eyes as she explained that faith wasn't something tangible like that. It was part of the mystery of Christ. It is what makes Christ real. It wasn't something you read in a book, but something that you experience. She assured me that the Holy Spirit was living in me and would help and guide me as I was seeking God for truth and understanding. She said Christ was just something she knew in her heart and that I would one day know that also. She was so confident in telling me that Christ was always with me and was watching over me every day and loved me, just because I was His daughter.

I still get strength from these words in times when I feel lost and confused by this world.

Mom was sensitive to others' needs. She always had a lot of friends. She sat down with them sharing hopes and dreams, passions and fears, heartache and wounds. She did things with Dad and other couples also. They were part of a group that had

Life Growing Up

"secret couples." Secret couples are like a secret Santa would be during Christmas time, but it lasted throughout the entire year. I have vivid memories of her making something special for the couple and decorating it as cute as could be. She would drop one of us kids off at the edge of the couple's house with the treat. We would sneak to the front door, place the item down, ring the doorbell, and run away as fast as we could out of sight. Mom and Dad got such joy out of giving. They lived out what Luke writes about in Acts 20:35 In everything I did, I showed you that by this kind of hard work we must help the weak, remembering the words the Lord Jesus himself said: 'It is more blessed to give than to receive.' Mom purposefully looked for ways to brighten up someone's day. She honestly did get more joy out of giving than receiving.

In high school, I tried out for the cheerleading squad. In the middle of the day, there was a call on the intercom for me to stop by the office between classes. With much nervous anxiety, I entered the office door to be presented with a vase of flowers from Mom to wish me luck for the tryouts after school. That's the kind of person she was, thoughtful and loving.

Sometimes, I was selfish and didn't always understand her generosity towards others. It became expected that there would be a guest at the dinner table on holidays. It took me a while to appreciate why she would invite someone that wasn't part of our family to participate in this special time with us. God always put someone on her heart that needed to be with a family on these special occasions. She opened her home as much as her heart to all that needed family and need to be loved. She believed we are all part of God's family.

Through my teen years, mom helped out at church during the week. She supported many different projects and programs the church held. She served in leadership roles in our Church

An Introspective Journey

Parish and helped plan the Sunday liturgy for Mass. She taught classes for youth and chaperoned numerous events. We knew that if mom wasn't at home or at work, she was probably at church. When the doors were open, we were there.

Her faith grew as she studied the Word more. Her relationship with Christ was intimate. Similarly, in the same way she interacted with close friends, she interacted with Christ. Somewhere in the late 1980s, she began writing in a prayer journal as a reflection of daily scripture. When we cleaned her house in 2015, we found 30 years of journal writings.

These journals were personal and private. It was here that she poured out her deepest thoughts, worries, fears, joys, secrets and embarrassing moments. She was able to more fully explore the meaning behind the scriptures and how it applied to the world around her through her journal writing. She encountered God, not by just dissecting the scripture, but by experiencing Him as she let Him into her soul. Mom knew she could never "figure out God" and didn't try to.

She describes it by saying,

It is amazing that the more you know about Jesus, the more there is to know. The more I know about Jesus the more I know about myself, the more I appreciate and love God. In my lifetime I will never know all there is to know about God nor will I know all there is to know about me. With God's revelation and with my openness to that, I will always find or uncover new things until I'm in heaven.

She routinely wrote about the comfort and peace she experienced always having a hunger for more of Christ. Here are some of her journal writings. Her prayers are vivid, as if Christ was right beside her.

Life Growing Up

7/10/1990
Mark 4:40
> He said to his disciples, "Why are you so afraid? Do you still have no faith?"

His words "Did you not have faith" struck me hard because even now I continue to hold back my trust in my attitude and actions. I cried on and off during this prayer time. First because of shame for my mistrust and then joy for the calm within that came during my prayer. The pink/red mist that surrounded me, the presence of my God, so powerful, so loving, telling me again to live each moment with the awareness of Him. Telling me to trust his guidance. Lord, help me to retain this calmness and abandonment to you. Amen.

8/6/1990
Prayer: Lord, you know me and you hold me; what comfort. You know my innermost fears and you love me. I am the doubter. I get so wrapped up in myself, I forget to let your work come through. How wonderful to be able to reach my arms out and you hold my weeping heart. You will not let me be harmed. You will always provide me with the right shield. I need only watch and listen. Thank you for the sunshine. Amen.

9/17/1990
I tried to abandon my thoughts and I saw a new daybreak. I was sitting in the open in a pasture on a hill or mountain. I knew this is the beginning of something new in my life, my spiritual life. After I sat for a while in the brightness of day. The wind began and a strong dust storm. Next, I was underwater (very blue). Then the blue turned to a bright green and I was in a tall meadow. Just like the cycles of growth in my vision. I started

to cry, but not for long. It was the Father who was showing me all this. I know He will always be with me no matter what I go through. I feel loved by God and everyone.

As years went on, she kept writing. Her writings included more than just an analysis of what was happening in Jesus' day, but how the scripture applied to her life personally. God was real to her in her prayer time.

More than once, she describes how she feels Jesus with her. Christ spoke to her in her prayer time and she journaled about her reactions.

The gift of Scripture is that it's not stagnant. It's a living word. It speaks to us differently each time. Because we are changed/different from the last time; the living word of God—Gift.

I was happy today to just sit with my Lord. Here, today, now, as I sat, I felt the presence of a hand in mine. I know that wherever I go or do that hand will always be there. How wonderful to never be alone. To be alone with God is never lonely nor is it crowded.

Job 1:21
> Naked I came from my mother's womb, and naked I will depart. The Lord gave and the Lord has taken away may the name of the Lord be praised.

All is a gift. I am accountable to God for the use of his gifts. Since all is gift, I need to appreciate every gift, not just the ones I feel are significant. Jesus sat with me and put his hand in mine. I became aware of something in my hand. I thought I was holding my own hands, but I wasn't. It was as if he said "I always hold your hand." I am so grateful for this time of prayer. I am loved so much! I feel so full of joy, so special, happy.

Life Growing Up

John 15:1-8

> I am the true vine, and my Father is the gardener. He cuts off every branch in me that bears no fruit, while every branch that does bear fruit he prunes so that it will be even more fruitful. You are already clean because of the word I have spoken to you. Remain in me, as I also remain in you. No branch can bear fruit by itself; it must remain in the vine. Neither can you bear fruit unless you remain in me.
>
> I am the vine; you are the branches. If you remain in me and I in you, you will bear much fruit; apart from me you can do nothing. If you do not remain in me, you are like a branch that is thrown away and withers; such branches are picked up, thrown into the fire and burned. If you remain in me and my words remain in you, ask whatever you wish, and it will be done for you. This is to my Father's glory, that you bear much fruit, showing yourselves to be my disciples.

John 15: 16-17

> You did not choose me. Instead, I chose you. I appointed you so that you might go and bear fruit that will last. I also appointed you so that the Father will give you what you ask for. He will give you whatever you ask for in my name. Here is my command. Love one another.

The main thing I think of today was my feeling of distance, the branch of a tree moves out from the vine or main trunk. I long to be close and next to the vine. I spoke to Jesus and told him I needed a hug. He gave me a hug. I cried a lot in this prayer period and I had a strong reluctance to end it. At one point I had a sensation of falling. Actually, my body jumped. It was pure reflex. Whatever happened was very strong. I wish I would have had the awareness to let myself go. I am sure it was God bringing me down somewhere and I did not allow it to happen.

Her journaling became very important to her. On a trip when she didn't have her journal she later writes,

I did not realize how much I depend on my journal for reflecting on my life. On our first morning here I awoke wanting to share my feelings. I felt lost without my friend the journal. It is also a very tangible representation of my conversations with Jesus. I truly felt a part of me was missing.

Matthew 25: 35-36
> I was hungry and you fed me, thirsty and you gave me a drink; I was a stranger and you received me in your homes, naked and you clothed me; I was sick and you took care of me, in prison and you visited me.

August 2005, Mom and Dad went above and beyond what many would be willing to do.

The city of New Orleans was being evacuated due to Hurricane Katrina. Her church called her and explained how the priests had been evacuated to a nearby retreat center. The bus driver and his family needed a place to stay. Of course, Mom and Dad opened their home to this family of strangers. This family was further devastated when they realized their home in New Orleans was completely destroyed and they were suddenly homeless. Mom and Dad provided for them in so many ways, more than just shelter and food, but emotionally supporting them during this tragic time, spiritually in prayer, and practically in helping them find a place to go. This was not easy. This family had special needs and unbeknown to us, her family, she had begun struggling with her memory. Her journal reflection on what was happening at the time of this tragedy expresses her heart.

My Jesus, what a call to love your brother. In this day and time, it can be life threatening. On a broad scale, this looting and disregard for life in this storm speaks of this. How many times have we said when we see another heading to trouble, "I'm not getting involved," "It's none of my business?" Where does our responsibility begin and end? It does not end until you have done all you can do.

When I began college in 1986, Mom decided it was time for her to also go back to school. She was 45 years old, but would not let that stop her. She received her Associates Degree in General Studies in December 1987, and then her Bachelor's Degree in May 1989. She didn't quit there. She pursued her studies at Loyola University and was awarded with a Master's Degree in Pastoral Studies in August 1993.

It was then that I believe she lived out her calling in its fullest. She worked at several churches as Director of Religious Education then moved into the Diocesans Office serving not just one church, but many. Her heart was big and wanted to share what she could following the call on her life. During this time, she even collaborated on a book setting up a curriculum for the RCIA Program (Rite of Christian Initiation of Adults). This program is designed for adult prospective converts to Catholicism. The candidates are gradually introduced to aspects of Catholic beliefs and practices.

An Introspective Journey

Mom could talk about the Bible and the history of the church with the best of them as well as debate on it, and she did. But more importantly was the example she set for all around her. She lived love. Her heart and home was always open. She was involved in so many different service projects and work for the Lord. But if someone knocked on the door or called her (and many did) she took time out of her busy schedule to visit with them. No one was ever turned away.

Chapter 3

CAREGIVING

As the years went on, Mom's parents required more and more help. Mom went with them to doctor visits and tried monitoring their medicines. She noticed them struggling with everyday life. Mom made sure to call them every day. More than once their phone rang and rang without an answer. They lived 45 minutes away from Mom and Dad. Mom would call their kind neighbor to check on them. Almost always they had simply not hung the phone up.

Then one day, her mother, Lucy, at 75 years old, suffered a stroke. Unbeknown to Mom at the time, her life changed forever on this day. The caregiving intensified as she knew her parents needed more help than she could give to them 45 minutes away. During this time was when Grandmother was officially diagnosed with Alzheimer's Disease. We all had an idea of what that would mean, or at least we thought we did. Many members from both sides of Mom's family (maternal and paternal) had struggled or were struggling with this disease. But no one can entirely be prepared for this disease. No one case is the same, but all cases are heartbreaking.

As Grandmother was recovering from her stroke in a rehab

facility, the comforting words from Isaiah became visibly apparent to Mom and Dad.

Isaiah 41:10
> So do not fear, for I am with you; do not be dismayed,
> for I am your God. I will strengthen you and help you;
> I will uphold you with my righteous right hand.

Dad was outside mowing his lawn when his neighbor stopped to visit. The neighbor told Dad of he and his wife's decision to move to another state to be closer to their family. Imagine the surprise this couple had when Dad offered to buy their house right then and there before it even came on the market. God provides when we don't have the answer. Time and time again we find He is at work when we are at wit's end.

Devotion

Isaiah 54:10-12
> Though the mountains be shaken and the hills be removed, yet my unfailing love for you will not be shaken nor my covenant of peace be removed," says the LORD, who has compassion on you. "O afflicted city, lashed by storms and not comforted, I will build you with stones of turquoise, your foundations with sapphires. I will make your battlements of rubies, your gates of sparkling jewels, and all your walls of precious stones.

We all have storms in our lives. Times we feel we are being

tossed back and forth on wild waves of life wondering how we can survive. Fear and anxiety can easily take over and consume us. We doubt where God is and when, or if, relief will come. Christ is like the lighthouse that is in the distance. It is what we see as the waves crash in our faces. The light guides our way to safety. We can lose our focus in the rough waters but must keep our eyes on the light, our eyes toward Christ, so He can rescue us. We want peace, we want it to stop. It is when we lean on Christ that He can carry us and provide for us through the storms in our lives. It is in these times, we can more fully surrender and let the Holy Spirit bring calm in the storm.

It was not difficult to convince Grandmother and Granddaddy to purchase the house next door in order for them to be better cared for. Mom and Dad were clever in putting together an alert system for when my grandparents needed help. They set up an emergency doorbell for them. When they needed help, all they had to do was to ring the doorbell that was located in their bedroom. The doorbell rang in Mom and Dad's house. Now when the doorbell rang, someone headed next door to help them. This worked well for a few years. Mom took them where they needed to go, cooked when she could and helped them keep their house clean.

Grandmother still tried cooking. After all, that is what she did best. Grandmother's food was "the best." This is where I noticed the first signs from Grandmother's illness. She went from being the "best cook" to her food being undercooked or overcooked. The foods she put together just didn't belong together. The amount of salt in her food made the food inedible. Their favorite food now was Bush's Baked beans from a can. It was about the only thing they ate that was worth eating. Arrangements were made for "Meals on Wheels" to be delivered at lunchtime. Mom provided their dinner meal. We knew how bad her cooking must have been when Grandmother and Granddaddy talked about "Meals on Wheels" being the best food ever. It was so much better than what they had been eating.

Their needs were becoming greater and greater. Something was finally done when Granddad fell and broke his hip. Grandmother needed 24-hour care and Granddad couldn't help. The decision was made to place them in a nursing home. Mom's brothers struggled with this action. Was this move going to sink them faster into the final stages of life or is this move going to provide for them what they need? Grandmother and Granddaddy went along with it because they thought it was temporary while Granddad healed from his broken hip. I believe the broken hip was a gift from God, nudging us to put them where they needed to be. At the nursing home, they thrived. Color came back to their faces and they smiled more often. They were around others, visited, played bingo, danced and even had parties. It was such a change from them being alone, without proper food or limited visitors.

Since Mom lived in town, she was the one who visited daily, took care of all the financial obligations, doctor visits, as well as their now vacant home. It was her responsibility. She did all this while still working full time and being involved in her community. What a strong woman she was. I watched all this as it happened, but never truly understood how hard it was on her to manage everything she was doing.

Her dad also had some dementia issues, although not specifically diagnosed as Alzheimer's. Even as Mom dealt with her parent's illnesses, she was beginning to realize she was also experiencing symptoms from this dreaded disease taking hold of her.

Caregiving

She prays in her journal:

My Jesus, give me the insight I need to do what is best for my parents and for myself and for Paul. I trust! Amen.

It isn't easy being a caregiver. It carries an emotional strain. Mom shares her raw feelings with her God.

My Lord and my God, there are so many areas of my life that need healing. I get so caught up in my own mire. I get stuck. I wallow in ingratitude. I miss the gift of you, my God. Perhaps the anger I feel when Dad begins bad mouthing and complaining triggers that part of me too. Before I can be grateful for the large things in my life, I must recognize those small, unseen burrows that wear away at my peace. There is so much disorder in my world. My job is to keep focused on the God who loves and calls me to love. Amen.

Devotion

I also feed on the emotions of others. I lose my perspective and lose sight of the small blessings that do come each day. The blessing of family, the blessing of time spent with them. The sunshine, my health. When I think about it, the list of blessings goes on and on. I must remind myself to center my eyes, my life, on Christ. God is good and wants to shower me with blessings. I just don't see it all the time. I see others and wonder why things are so good for them. I question, why do things go well for everyone else, but me? I convince myself no one else has to struggle like I do. I believe no one hurts the way I do. I am so sure that no one understands. I think everyone else's life is better than mine.

An Introspective Journey

I ask, "why?" But that isn't the truth. My attitude is what determines my actions. I have a choice to look at the positive or look at the negative. We live in a world where bad things happen. But we also live in a world where I can make a difference. I can make a difference to those I come in contact with. No matter how difficult my life becomes, I can influence others.

What will my influence be? Will I point to the hope that Christ offers? Will I encourage others not to give up? Will I make a difference in the lives of those that struggle through heartache and diseases?

Christ does not promise everything will be perfect. We grow in our struggles. Mom made people happy when she was with them. She followed Christ's command to "Love each other as I have loved you." (John 15:12)

As mom continues to care for her parents she writes more of the struggle that comes from being a caregiver.

Oct. 22, 2001

My Jesus, for a long time things have been gnawing at me, my resentment for the burdens placed on me for my parents. I know I am insensitive to their pain because I am so caught up in my own. It affects all that I do. My Jesus, forgive me. Give me the grace to forgive myself. Help me to let go of the past and to live in the present, the what is now, and you are here with me. Let me forgive myself.

Romans 8:6

> The concerns of the flesh is death, but the concerns of the Spirit is life and peace.

Caregiving

My Jesus, how wonderful is your love. Those little touches to let me know that you are with me. As I sat here in reflection I felt the heaviness of the concerns of the flesh, the darkness, the limiting of hope. Oh, but, what joy when I felt the infusion of light and peace. It was definitely a grace-filled moment bringing tears. When now, as I reflect, My Jesus, help me remember that joy and love throughout my day. Thank you, my Lord and my God, my friend. Love, Bev.

Grandmother's progression in the disease was evident. If something happened, such as a fall or illness, a bit more of her memory would leave her never to return. One day when I was visiting her she asked, "Who are you?"

I answered, "Paula, Beverly's daughter."

She looked at me questionably. All she could say was, "But Beverly's not married."

How do you respond to that? From that time on, Mom asked everyone to no longer call her "Grandmother," but instead to call her "Lucy." She was confused by the name, Grandmother. We'd sit in her room as she told us stories of long ago as if they were happening at that moment. The disease crept into so many areas of her life. When she forgot how to stand up from a chair, the nurses tried to teach her the process to no avail. She no longer talked, but when Christmas time came around, could sing some of the songs with the music. There were times she would grab in the air and move her fingers in a particular pattern. We tried to figure out what she might be doing in her mind. To this day, we don't know, but we suspect she was either saying her rosary or cleaning beans out of their shells like she had done for many years with the beans from their garden.

In this phase of Mom's life, she prepared for the future that lurked ahead. Spiritually, she was learning to gain strength from

An Introspective Journey

her heavenly Father. God showed his faithfulness by always providing her love and peace, even on difficult days.

With caring for her parents, Mom knew all too well the strain that comes from this disease and the toll it puts on family members both financially and emotionally. It was during this time she and Dad purchased long term care insurance. Dad has said multiple times that this was the best thing they ever did. Because of this wise purchase, we, the family, are not financially burdened and Mom is able to get the care she needs.

As Mom made decisions regarding her parents, she would tell us, "When this happens to me, do such and such." Or "Don't let me do this or that." She wanted to live with dignity and not be a burden to anyone.

As much as I didn't want any of those things to happen, they still did. When they happened, she didn't have rational thoughts and actions to accept her earlier wishes. She simply could not comprehend where she was in her mind. When confronted with things she was saying or doing, she didn't believe what we said was true. She thought we were making things up. She believed people were out to get her. She was determined and did what she thought was correct in the way her mind told her it was.

It's a strange way to view things. To watch her make such odd decisions and do such unusual things, knowing how opposite it would be if she had been in her right mind. Her actions turned oppositional. Her composition was sluggish and saddened. She was in inner turmoil and paranoid, so her trust in anyone and everyone was compromised.

When caring for Mom was no longer possible in her home, it was our conversations from when she cared for her parents that gave us confidence in knowing we were making the right decision. It was her own words, stated years earlier, that rang in our ears. We knew her wishes. She didn't want to be a burden to anyone or to change their life around for her sake, to care for her. At the same time, she wanted to have as much independence as possible but mostly she still wanted to be loved and not forgotten. We don't have to live with worry or guilt for placing her in the care of others. She never revolted in the way we feared. We found a facility that was caring and compassionate. They truly love her, despite her disease. In her heart, I believe she knew we were doing what was best for her. Perhaps that's why she has always been kind in accepting the care from the facilities where she lived.

It is in her journals that we discovered how long Mom struggled with the symptoms of Alzheimer's Disease and how she chose to deal with it. Most of her writings ended in 2009, although she had a few in 2010 when the disease had taken away her ability to put together her thoughts and write it down. Her earliest writing expressing her disease came in the year 1999 when she was 57 years old. She wonders if this might be Alzheimer's Disease.

Chapter 4

THE EARLY YEARS OF ALZHEIMER'S

12/30/1999

Thank you my Jesus for the journey and your constant companionship. Without it I would not be here. Continue to be my protector and my devil's advocate. Give me clarity in those very cloudy times, where I have lost my direction. Your love and grace is all I need. I love you Lord. Amen.

2/23/00

Lord, if I may ask, please help me with remembering. Is it that I cannot relax? Is it something physical? ...That dreaded "A" word? Whatever it is, give me the strength of your love. Amen.

Devotion

What a question to have to ask yourself. How do individuals

react when they initially believe they may have Alzheimer's? Sometimes news is too terrible to believe. Why don't we believe certain things? Privately, Mom did come to realize she had Alzheimer's, but she never would say out loud that she suffered from this disease. Maybe if she didn't believe it, others wouldn't believe either. Maybe if she said it out loud, it would become more real. She wanted to hide from this disease, wanting to overcome and live a normal life. In doing so, she was also convinced that the things we told her she was saying and doing were not true. She denied so much. Was it perhaps too terrible to believe she would act and say the things she did?

What are we in denial about? The way we perceive something is the way we act, how we respond to others. Am I trying to hide from the truth of some circumstance in my life? I need to listen when loved ones caution me about things I say and do. I ask the Wonderful Counselor, to guide my steps and thoughts into the reality I face. When I face reality, I can move forward in my situation. I also ask the Prince of Peace to come to my aid. I admit it, I can't handle life with all the circumstances I face on my own.

Join me with Mom on her journey through scripture and prayer. As you get to know my mom, also grow in understanding the years of struggle for someone living with Alzheimer's Disease. Grow spiritually in surrender to God, regardless of the outcome.

3/7/00
Genesis 1:27
    So God created mankind in his own image, in the

image of God he created them; male and female he created them.

What a challenge "to describe myself in just 2 words"— Determination and open minded. It seems I want to do this in terms of my feelings. Perhaps my feelings are determined by what I am. All I know is that I am tired of feeling "out of it." I don't really know what I'm supposed to be about. I don't know how to regain myself assurance.

10/26/00

My Jesus, so much of what I want is in the moment. I desire to have some longevity of thought and continuity. These memory problems scare me to death. Just the fear of it is beginning to inhibit me. Help me Jesus to be more alert and mindful. Help me Jesus. I am afraid.

She continues her struggle within herself trying to stay focused in her confusion:

11/27/2000

Your constant and unconditional love, my Lord, has sustained me thus far in my confusion and in my inertia. Sustained me and lead me into a peaceful garden. Why is it hard? Turmoil and unrest plague me. I can't seem to just be without something that I should be doing. Why do I take on so much responsibility? When will I sort out the necessary from the life that can go on without me? Thank you Lord for the little embrace a minute ago. Continue to lead me to your work and to the kingdom. Thank you for the peace. Amen!

THE EARLY YEARS OF ALZHEIMER'S

Devotion

Psalm 55:22
>Cast your cares on the Lord and he will sustain you; he will never let the righteous be shaken.

God's word says he will sustain me. It doesn't say he might sustain me, but he will. I also have times of turmoil and unrest. Do I question if Christ will sustain me or do I just hope things will work out? Do I really believe that Christ is in my life and wanting to help me through this? And if he does, why doesn't He just take the pain away? Do I unintentionally create a barrier or obstacle to Christ helping me because I am trying to be strong and deal with it on my own? I will remember what Mom did as she looked for small reassurances from God that He is doing as He promised and sustain me in my times of distress. I will learn to take the focus off of me and instead put the focus on Christ.

11/28/2000

My Jesus, I worry about my ability to focus to move forward and sometimes not move at all, even retreating. What is wrong with me? Help me Lord accomplish my tasks. Help me to have that joy for life I used to have. I know I am loved by you. I'm just not sure how to respond at times. Am I following your will for me? Bring back my joy. Amen.

A few months go by as her struggle continues to haunt her.

She doesn't know how to describe it but refers to it as her disease.

1/15/2001
Matthew 13:1

> He replied, "Because the knowledge of the secrets of the kingdom of heaven has been given to you, but not to them."

"To enter into the deep Mystery of God"! My God, I long for your presence. My heart and soul long for you, my God. But the flesh is weak. Strengthen me, my Lord, to know and understand your presence in my world. Take away the laziness, the procrastination. Teach me your ways my Lord. I long for the peace I once had within and in my life. HELP!

1/16/2001

My Jesus, I am so messed up, confused, fearful, lost. I hate what I am becoming. I long for peace of heart and mind. Help me, my God! I am lost. I again ask for this cup to be taken. What I need is the courage and grace to do what needs to be done and set limits for myself and to move forward and not retreat into nothing. Help me, my Jesus. I need structure! Thanks for this time of quiet. Amen.

Devotion

Quiet time is underrated. I rush around life multi-tasking to get things done. Too often my life is measured by how much

I can do in a certain period of time. There's so little time to be quiet. So little time to "Be still and know that I am God." (Psalm 46:10) It is in time spent with Jesus that I begin to realize how deep and wide His love for me really is. It is in spending time with Him, I learn to live in my circumstances. This is when I begin to appreciate the beauty around me and see the blessings He has given me.

All this requires quiet time to allow Christ to enter peace into my troubled mind and heart. It allows Christ to help me distinguish what's important and what is not. It is here that I gain that courage to do what needs to be done and to follow God's will for my life.

1/19/2001
Jeremiah 31:33

> "This is the covenant I will make with the people of Israel after that time," declares the Lord. "I will put my law in their minds and write it on their hearts. I will be their God, and they will be my people."

My Lord, you have a wonderful way of reminding and connecting things for me. Is this not similar/or the cause of discernment of spirits? Thank you, my Lord, for the disease that happens within me to cause me to re-evaluate my life and my actions. Keep me safe today. Amen.

1/29/2001

Loving Lord, Show me the way to peace and tranquility. I long for inner quiet.

Devotion

We all have times of trials, times we feel lost, times in the wilderness. We have a choice. We can become bitter and angry. But there is a better way, although it is hard. We can't fall into the trap of questioning God's provision in our life. Life can stink and can drag us down. We must remember things we are thankful for instead of letting our struggles consume us. I must remember my testimony, remember what Christ has already brought me through. Let's be thankful together. Begin by finding at least 3 new things each day you are grateful for. Maybe it is just that you have breath, maybe it is the sunrise, or that you have food to eat or a place to lay your head. There is always something to be thankful for. Share your thankfulness with someone each day. What might our day look like if our thankful sharing leads others to also be thankful?

The intensity of her life is bottled up. She describes how she is feeling, but can't put a name to it. She learns to lean on Christ to get her through.

3/13/2001

My Jesus, I struggle so hard to find peace. The tranquility I do have will be shattered soon it seems. Please help me be Christ-like in my attitudes and behavior. Give me peace in this situation. Help me my Jesus in this situation and with my studies, and my job. I feel so scattered much of the time. My memory is very poor. I am frightened by this. Teach me courage and perseverance. Help me to learn my limitations and to be committed to what I can and not what I cannot.

3/25/2001

My Jesus, I am fearful of so many things, my ability to do my job, my relationship with my children, my ability as a Spiritual Director. Most of all I question "me." How do I love? Do I give my all? Why not? What do I fear? You, my Jesus, gave all. Teach me how to hold on to courage and to do what is hard, but what is right. Teach me to love beyond myself to help another. Help me to find peace in this present situation. Help me to forgive myself and others. Be with me Lord, let me see your face in all I encounter. I long for tranquility. I love you my God Help me to love better. Amen.

Devotion

Doesn't Jesus demand we give our all to Him? If God expects unconditional surrender, what does that look like in real life? Perhaps that is what Paul is talking about in Romans 12:1 "Therefore, I urge you, brothers and sisters, in view of God's mercy, to offer your bodies as a living sacrifice, holy and pleasing to God—this is your true and proper worship."

This scripture calls me to be a living sacrifice. Living implies life. Life is every day, in every relationship, every responsibility, every occasion, every success, and every failure. It is demonstrated by how I live, what I say, where I go, and what I do. When I allow Christ to be alive in me, I become more like him. I must pray for my thoughts to be Christ's thoughts and my actions His actions. I must never forget whose I am, and who I represent. It is when my focus leaves Christ and falls on me that I falter. I continually must be renewed, because I am imperfect. All I can do is to give the best I can in the best way I can and the God who is all knowing will always respond with mercy and grace.

Time continues and she writes in other entries such things as "I am afraid to lose me." And "I feel lost so often. Help me!" She has times she feels the presence of God and thanks him for "the gift of things being calming and peaceful." She thanks God for being able to focus, noting how long it has been since she was able to focus. She explains more of what she is experiencing and how she finds strength and hope through scripture.

5/2001
Joshua 3:3

>   You will leave your position and follow it, so that you may know which way to take, since you've never been that way before.

Yes, Lord. I have been struggling knowing which way to go. It seems I want to go in every direction. I am easily attracted to new things to do, but, I also want to continue the other things. I am finding myself becoming paralyzed because of the intensity of my life.

Help me Lord, give me the strength and the insight to unclutter my life. I am not sure what it looks like right now in my life. Show me or give me the grace to live in ambiguity. Continue to call me Lord, please don't give up on me. I am wandering in the desert. I feel lost so often. Help me! Amen.

Devotion

Do you ever feel as if you wander in the desert? Time in the desert and the wilderness is uncomfortable. So why do we remain there so long? We can choose to stay in the desert or look toward the Promised Land. We have a choice.

2 Corinthians 4:17 "For our light and momentary troubles are achieving for us an eternal glory that far outweighs them all."

This scripture tells us me I have something to look forward to. God is taking me somewhere. He is taking you somewhere too. God wants the best for us. He wants more for me than I can comprehend.

He has a bright future for me and for you. In Exodus, Moses is taking the Israelites to the Promised Land. They wandered in the desert for 40 years. It wasn't meant to be that long. This trip was only supposed to be a few months of traveling. It was longer because of the choices the people made. Am I wandering in the desert longer than I should be? Can I accept what is happening in my life and then look forward to the hope that Christ had promised me?

6/18/2001

My Jesus, help me to understand what is going on in my subconscious. Those episodes of what seem to be reality. Lord, give me the insight and the strength to understand and repair whatever is happening in my head. I am frightened. Help me Lord, for I am in trouble.

6/27/2001
Isaiah 40:31

> But those who hope in the Lord will renew their strength. They will soar on wings like eagles; they will run and not grow weary, they will walk and not be faint.

Father God, for so long I have felt like I am holding on to a thread, holding on for dear life! I know I can't go back to how things were and don't want to, but the future is vague, uncertain. The word "hope" is so encouraging. It has recurred several times this week in my prayer. Hope gives me a promise, a promise that you are always with me loving me, because of who you are not because of who I am. The promise is that I am always loved by you. I am not always lovable, but I am always loved. How wonderful. You are my God!

There are times she feels she can overcome:

7/22/2001
Matthew 4:6

> "If you are the Son of God," he said, "throw yourself down. For it is written: "He will command his angels concerning you, and they will lift you up in their hands, so that you will not strike your foot against a stone."

On this particular day, this scripture is making me uncomfortable. I "throw myself down" when I neglect my responsibilities when I procrastinate; make excuses for my own laziness. I sell my soul to the devil in so many subtle ways. The grace my Lord, to take control and to take responsibility with you at my side all is possible.

Show me your way. For me, I have felt lost for some time, in a partial haze. The clouds are clearing. Please, my friend, continue to call me out. I am grateful or this time. With all my love, Bev

Devotion

Whatever you're going to do, do it now. Don't say, "Tomorrow, next week, next month, or next year." It's now or never. Seize the moment! Every day, there are opportunities all around for a fresh start, but am I taking advantage of them? Why? One word: procrastination. Procrastination is strange. It's as if I think it will make my life easier when in reality it usually creates more stress. The truth is, I already know the right things to do and the benefits of doing the right things in life.

So why don't I do them? I do it all the time. For instance, why do I wait until evening to read my Bible when I know full well that I will be too tired to read or concentrate then? The Bible warns us there is no guarantee for tomorrow. Jesus said, "No procrastination. No backward looks. You can't put God's kingdom off till tomorrow. Seize the day" (Luke 9:62 MSG). I do it so unintentionally. I innocently do not even think about it. Perhaps I need to pray about what areas or situations I need to stop procrastinating. Maybe even ask myself what would I want to accomplish today if I knew tomorrow would not come.

Mom is touched by a prayer "Take and Receive." She surrenders.

An Introspective Journey

Suscipe

St. Ignatius of Loyola

> Take, Lord, and receive all my liberty,
> my memory, my understanding,
> and my entire will,
> all I have and call my own.
> You have given all to me.
> To you, Lord, I return it.
> Everything is yours; do with it what you will.
> Give me only your love and your grace,
> that is enough for me.

9/2001

My Jesus, what emotion evolved from the "Take and Receive" prayer.

Take my memory, understanding... If I had to choose a faculty that I would not want to lose is memory and understanding. Yet, Lord, you may call me to that. Am I willing to surrender? Yet, Lord, I know you will love and care for me in any state of mind or condition. If that would be what will be asked of me, My God, help me to accept. Give me the grace of surrender to your will.

Love, Bev

Once again, Mom recognizes she cannot control everything. She tries to let go.

10/12/01

My Loving Lord, again you remind me that I am a loved sinner. So much of my energy is spent in hiding my inadequacies. So much of what I do is what I think others expect and a vision of how I think I should be. As I fall deeper and deeper into aging I want to maintain, "how things were" instead of dealing with "how things are." My ego continues to get in the way. But you have shown me, Lord, that I cannot control everything. I've known that for a long time, but I was afraid to let go. My life lately has been out of my control and I haven't been able to handle things to keep control of it. When I really need to let go I cannot control others and situations. My loving friend, Jesus, help me to let go. To trust in your will for me. Help me to surrender to your will and your love. —Amen

As Mom takes care of her aging parents, she struggles with her own issues.

11/2001

Be with me Lord, my emotions, my physical health is in trouble. You say "ask and you shall receive, seek and you shall find" Matthew 7:7
Help me to see you in all this transition with my parents. Lord, I put my life in your hands and Mom and Dad's life. I love you my Lord and my all. Bev

Deut. 30:14
>No, the word is very near you; it is in your mouth and in your heart so you may obey it.

This passage gives me confidence and courage. Again, I ask for you to carry me. I am scattered, disoriented, in my work and life right now. Put me together — carry me- lead me, walk with me. Amen.

Heb. 4:12-13

> For the word of God is alive and active. Sharper than any double-edged sword, it penetrates even to dividing soul and spirit, joints and marrow; it judges the thoughts and attitudes of the heart. Nothing in all creation is hidden from God's sight. Everything is uncovered and laid bare before the eyes of him to whom we must give account.

"The word of God is able to discern reflections and thought of the heart"

My Jesus, your words, the words of the Father challenge my way of thinking and doing. I am grateful for the disease and the examination of conscience that your words cause in me. I especially am grateful for those joyful inner touches that your word initiates within me. The tears of joy and sorrow. It is these that touches the heart of my soul — not the head but the heart. What a gift to know I am loved in spite of myself — and because of that love I can and do change — Love, Bev

Fear is her greatest emotion.

11/2001
Luke 19: 10
> The Lord God has come to save what was lost.

My Jesus, open my heart and my mind to the forgiveness, acceptance, and care that you are holding out to me. I realize today just how much I have lost. I have put a wall up to avoid my feelings. I do not feel anymore, at least not loving or positive feelings. I am always on the defensive. I am almost void of feelings. I can't even express them. "Fear" is probably the most frequent feeling. Fear because I am so forgetful. Fear because I'm apathetic. Even my self-esteem has just about disappeared. And the greatest fear is that of being found out that I will not be respected, and the fear of losing my mind. The other fear I have is that of not being able to be responsible and losing respect from others.

My Jesus, I want to do your will, but I think that I am trying to make my will your will for me. I pray for the grace of trust and abandonment to your will. Let your will be done not mine. Amen. Again my Lord, teach me to trust, be patient with me. I am lost! Come and find me. Amen.

Devotion

Can we really live a life free of fear? The Bible speaks to us about fear again and again. My mind knows the words, "Do not be anxious about anything."; "Do not fear."; "Be not afraid." My heart just doesn't seem to always listen or believe. I have to remind myself of the promise from God. I remind myself of all the times He has gotten me through trials. I remind myself of the miracles around me and the good things He has done. I need to remember that no matter how I feel, God is faithful and will always be with me. When times are uncertain, I fear. I then begin to rely on Christ that is within me and not on my own ability. It is in the pain and struggle that I am challenged to grow.

Mom was in a car accident. She didn't notice a car coming in her direction. No one was injured, but it frightened her. She is beginning to recognize her actions affect others.

An Introspective Journey

11/01
Hosea 14:4-5

>I will heal their waywardness and love them freely, for my anger has turned away from them. I will be like the dew to Israel; he will blossom like a lily. Like a cedar of Lebanon he will send down his roots.

Hosea 14:9

>Who is wise? Let them realize these things. Who is discerning? Let them understand. The ways of the Lord are right; the righteous walk in them, but the rebellious stumble in them.

My Lord, in your word, in your timing there are no accidents. The readings today are so comforting in view of yesterday's accident. I do feel lost, scattered, on another plane much of the time lately. Because of this preoccupation with "stuff" in my life I am responsible for the problems others will experience because of my distraction. I am so sorry. I take responsibility. Teach me the way to go. I realize I'm holding onto a string so much of the time. I'm afraid to let go. I am not alone. What happens will affect the life of another, Paul. Lord, help me to feel I am a good and loving and lovable person. Is this my own private emotional breakdown? Amen.

11/14/01
Anima Christi

>Jesus, may all that is in you flow into me.
>May your body and blood be my food and drink.
>May your passion and death be my strength and life.
>Jesus, with you by my side enough has been given.
>May the shelter I seek be the shadow of your cross.

The Early Years of Alzheimer's

Let me not run from the love which you offer.
But hold me safe from the forces of evil.
On each of my dyings shed your light and your love.
Keep calling to me until that day comes.
When with our saints, I may praise you forever. Amen.

David Fleming, S.J.

"May the shelter I seek be the shadow of your cross"
My Jesus, I am overwhelmed by this verse, this prayer. The shadow is shelter. It is a conduit of the father's love. A place of comfort, a place of being "there" and not have to do anything for the gift. Jesus earned it for me. Lord, the emotion is giving me release; perhaps just as you released in "commending your spirit" on the cross. Continue to be so obvious in your love for me. I need a lot of TLC. I am so afraid with this short memory. I love you my Jesus. Bev

Prayers for healing of emotions.

11/17/01

My Jesus, I am paralyzed by fear, anxiety, anger, jealousy, by the need to be loved and liked. I so wish to be healed. Many times I feel like the man on the pallet, helpless. (Mark 2:1-12) Who will love me enough to go to the extreme for my healing? Paul has already done this for me a thousand times. When will I get up and walk on my own? Heal me my Lord and God my friend. Amen.

Prayers for refuge.

11-28-01
Isaiah 1:8

And daughter Zion is left like a hut in a vineyard,
like a shed in a melon patch, like a city blockade.

My Lord, in the midst of the turmoil the pain the fear, the insecurity, the uncertainty, you are my refuge, shelter from the storm. Today my Lord, I ask for the strength for my day. To be focused and productive. You are my refuge. Be my strength today! Love, Bev

Future uncertain.

12/26/01

...I want to be loved just for me. Otherwise, I have no worth at all. When I can't do anymore, will I be discarded, forgotten? Lord, be with me in my pain....

Devotion

One of our most basic fundamental needs is to be loved. God is love. (I John 4:8) No one can show the unconditional love the way our Father has for us. To truly love, we must first understand God's love. And accept it unconditionally. We tend to judge rather harshly. We expect perfection, from ourselves and others. We believe others also expect perfection. The mind is a powerful tool. When I think negative thoughts, my actions show it. The way I view myself has an impact on the way others see me. If I believe I have no worth, I will begin acting that way and, consequently, others will believe it also.

Am I only loved and valued when I am productive? Christ

says NO! Letting our minds linger in this filth will rob us from opportunities to experience joy in all circumstances. Christ desires to lavish me in his love.

I John 3:1
> See what great love the Father has lavished on us, that we should be called children of God! And that is what we are! The reason the world does not know us is that it did not know him.

Mom struggles with her anger being born of fear. She writes about times of feeling unaccepted, unloved, scattered and lost. She asks God to center her back to the love and mission. She thanks God for her friends. She continues to pray for life again, memory and all. As the years progress, Mom begins to see her illness taking over her actions. She tries to make sense out of the inner turmoil she is experiencing.

1/12/02

My Jesus, I sit here joyful to be again in a quiet space for you and me. Again trust comes up. I do trust in your presence and in your guiding my journey. I also see how easily I can be distracted. Continue to call me back, to center me on your presence and your life within me on your presence and your life within my world and me. Lord, help me to know my limitations. Give me the grace to prepare well to present well the retreats you call me to. I am fearful. I do not trust myself. OK, Lord, it is not me but you who does the inspiring, challenging in retreats or in spiritual direction.

Devotion

God created each of us for a purpose. Our purpose is to be the clay in the potter's hand. (Isaiah 64:8) If God is the potter, then we were created to be molded and shaped into what pleases God. My purpose is to be a vessel for Christ. I have been commanded to spread the Good News. For Christ to use me, my vessel must be empty of selfishness and of worldly things I have placed there. Once it is empty, I have to be clean.

How can I be inspiring for others to follow Christ, if my life is dirty? Lastly, to be used by Christ I must desire to share. Our Lord never forces us. It is His desire to use us. It is when I empty myself, clean my life, and fill with His love that I am most effectively a servant spreading his message. I know I cannot serve Him alone. I can only do what I do for Him when I allow Him to guide my every step.

5/5/02

My Jesus, I so often am filled with inner turmoil. I can't seem to balance my activities. Sometimes I feel I am on the edge of emotion of feeling but I in some ways have put up a wall in fear of being hurt and disappointed. Yet, I keep trying to break through. To love and be loved without fear and without counting cost. I've been disappointed so many times that I fear I have never learned to love so I don't know how to respond to love. Teach me to give all of myself without counting cost. Let me imitate your way of loving and being. Jesus, my friend, Help me! Love, Bev

THE EARLY YEARS OF ALZHEIMER'S

Devotion

Matthew 12:29-30

> And everyone who has left houses or brothers or sisters or father or mother or wife or children or fields for my sake will receive a hundred times as much and will inherit eternal life. But many who are first will be last, and many who are last will be first.

This scripture is our call to perfect love. Before every meal and gathering, it was Mom's joy to lead us in prayer. She would always include the words, "Lord, make us better lovers of you." It sounds really great, and I'd think that's a neat idea, but never completely understood these words. How do we become better lovers of Christ? Hope is found through grace in the arms of Christ. When I am being held by the Almighty God and Father, I know I've been sought after and found. His embrace surrounds me with his love and protection and in his love and acceptance, he builds our dreams anew from the inside out. The truth is that I am infinitely more precious to God than he is to me. I'm accepted when I'm unacceptable and I'm loved when I am unlovable. After all these years, I think I finally understand her words. It isn't until we understand Jesus' perfect love can we then demonstrate that love to others. Oh, how I desire to be a better lover for Christ. Maybe instead of thinking of all my troubles, pay attention to what others are going through? Perhaps I'd give more time to sharing and listening to others. Could my words be kinder and more forgiving? Would I act differently if I saw myself the way Jesus sees me? He doesn't see what isn't, but rather what could be. He is always rooting for me and yet how often do I encourage others? I have a long way to go. Maybe more through what I have failed to do in addition to what I have done.

8/26/02

I long for an extended time of quiet and peace. A time without stress or demands. Teach me to find these moments. To recognize them and to make the best of them. My Jesus, I do feel that my life is changing. I have some fear of what might be. Bring me peace, walk with me into this unknown. Give me the grace of trust.

Mom served as caregiver for both of her parents. Her mother was also diagnosed with Alzheimer's Disease. Mom recognizes characteristics from her mother in herself.

9/2002
Psalm. 7:1
> Lord my God, I take refuge in you; save and deliver me from all who pursue me.

My Jesus the thought occurs to me that part of my struggle is allowing uncomfortable things to magnify into huge stresses. Much of my turmoil is my lack of coping skills, mechanisms. So many times, my Jesus, I am my own worst enemy. My resistance to face reality, to face the painful and the uncomfortable. I know in my head life is not a "bowl of cherries," but I try so hard to ignore the reality. Intersecting what I've seen so long ago and disliked in Momma, I'm seeing in myself. I am truly a fallen and forgiven sinner. Thank you my Lord—Amen.

Chapter 5

MOUNTING LIMITATIONS

4/07/2004

> "Guard my integrity when I am tempted to sell what is precious to my soul."
>
> Joyce Rupp

My Jesus, I had not seen my struggle. My dishonesty, my betrayal as I struggle with memory, but especially with depression and lethargy (in everything). It is only in coming through the fog can I see the magnitude of my deception; to myself and others. I was committing suicide in so many ways, especially with justification of my actions and attitudes.

I see even more clearly how suicide is such a selfish act. I have run away from the truth (reality) for a while—unwilling to face "what is." I have allowed that to color so much of my life. My Jesus, I have been Judas so often, yet, you forgive time after time. Your love is so constant.

What a gift to know that love. I am so grateful for the gift of recognition of my sinfulness. I can be like Judas so sure my way is "the way" that I compromise my integrity to accomplish "my right."

Forgive me, Lord.

Devotion

Haven't we all been Judas at one time or another? Don't we deny the will of Christ and do our will instead? The gift is recognizing our mistake and where that will lead us. Without acknowledging our sin, we can't receive forgiveness and turn back to Christ. Christ's love is so amazing that no matter where my sinfulness has taken me, He will always forgive when I ask for forgiveness with a repentant heart.

Peter also denied Jesus right after Judas did. The outcome for each was different. Peter knew of Christ's love and asked for forgiveness and became the rock on which the church began. Judas, on the other hand, never asked for forgiveness. His life ended by his own hand when he came to understand he had betrayed the Son of God. He couldn't live with this guilt. The sad news is that he didn't have to live with the guilt and shame. Jesus had the power to wipe away his sin, even the sin of betrayal. How often have I created an obstacle and have been unable to move forward because of my stubbornness in trying to fit God into my will instead of fitting my life into His will?

7/2004

My Jesus, I am grateful for this week. It has given me more energy for the kingdom. It has also given rise to my movement into the "autumn" of my life! I am not who I was, so present in my forgetting, but Lord, the possibilities of building the kingdom draws me. I believe you are the instrument of my movement to

Mounting Limitations

this place. I did not seek. The invitation was from beyond me. Help me always to be present to you, to trustingly discern your will for me. Amen.

11/2004
Isaiah 35:3-4

> Strengthen the feeble hands, steady the knees that give way; say to those with fearful hearts, 'Be strong, do not fear your God will come, he will come with vengeance, with divine retribution he will come to save you.'

My Jesus, I am fearful. Concerns for the future, concerns about my relationship with my family, concerns about my forgetfulness, concerns about this and that. I trust that you love me, Lord, but I don't always trust that my love for you is strong enough. I ask for the grace to trust that you will give me the gift of trust, the gift to recognize you in everything and everyone; to be grateful for your life in all of creation; in all the messiness of living. Teach me to love. Teach me how!!!!

Eventually, Mom realizes she has limitations. She struggles just to keep up day to day. Finding peace is paramount. It was during this time, she consulted her primary care physician. Her doctor did prescribe Aricept. She was very private about this medication and only told her family that she had "a little bit of dementia." It was many, many years before she mentioned aloud to anyone about her struggles with her memory. Her cries out to her God become more intense, wanting to serve, but plagued by this disease.

3/2005
Matthew 18:21-22

> Then Peter came to Jesus and asked, 'Lord, how

many times shall I forgive my brother or sister who sins against me? Up to seven times?' Jesus answered, 'I tell you, not seven times, but seventy-seven times.

My Jesus, I long for your peace within. I live my life in stress. Help me to know my limitations, to recognize my gifts and to be attentive to your presence. Teach me, Lord, to be honest within myself so that I can be honest and authentic with others. Give me the grace of memory. Lord, I am so very grateful for your love and presence. I love you my Jesus. I really push you on forgiving. 7 X 70 X ____. It is what keeps me going, your love and forgiveness. Love Bev

Devotion

God's grace is sufficient for me. I start with prevenient grace which is the grace that comes even before I came to recognize and follow Christ. Next, I look to justifying grace that leads me through reconciliation, forgiveness, and restoration; just as if I had never sinned. Lastly, I come to sanctifying grace. This grace goes on and on as I grow and mature in my Christian walk. I mature through the power of the Holy Spirit. Grace is always with me. It is a gift that's been given to help me in my life and situations daily. I'd be lost entirely without grace.

2005

In the autumn of my life, I am beginning to recognize the

Mounting Limitations

presence of God in the ordinary things, the everydayness of my life. I often think of that song "Looking for love in all the wrong places." Looking to be knocked off my horse so to speak. Happiness is in the quiet moments and in the ordinariness of my day. I need only to look around. Both of my parents have dementia. Their illness has helped me to be more in the present. To find the joy and presence of God in every moment. Happiness is an inside job. It comes from that original grace given to each of us when God breathes life into us.

11/2005

My Jesus, help me to know your will for me. I get so confused. I fear losing my mind. I long to be free of this state of confusion. I want to live in the moment, but the moment brings with it the past and the possibility of the future. I live in the moment, not remembering the past. I have no past, which gives me no anticipation for the future. I only have the present. This is so scary! Without past, how do I know who I am? Who am I? Help me Lord, to know, at least who I am in you. I hate this self-centeredness I've become. I want to do for others, yet I'm stuck in moment by moment. It is so hard to describe. I cannot do what I used to do. My Jesus, give me peace!

Devotion

How difficult it must be not to have a past to pull from. It would be as if everyone I spoke with were a stranger, even when I could say who they were. What would we talk about? No wonder conversation dies down. It's like there is a blank page that she felt obligated to fill up. That's why our conversations were so confusing and abruptly start and stop. I often live either in the future or the past. I seem to either reminisce or plan for the future. Perhaps I can try to live in the moment sometimes. Do I need to slow down and just be? Be with me Lord, be with my family, my friends and to be myself, no judging, no pretending, just be. It is when we are free to be truthful, letting go of the way I want them to be, that I can live in the moment of what Christ wants for me.

Knowing now how she is treating others disturb Mom. She prays not to bring pain to anyone due to her actions. She fears of not being loved.

11/2005

My Jesus, thank you for the time I had yesterday to get my work done and to be focused. Give me the grace of remembering all that I read and felt. I am afraid that my mind is leaving me. It is a constant reminder that we know not the future; that I am not in control of my destiny. I have only this moment! Help me Lord to be the best that I can be. Spare me Lord from bringing pain to anyone because of my disability. I long to know that I am truly loving self-giving person. However, my selfish nature continues to get in the way. I hate that part of me. That vision focuses on "me." Heal me of all that baggage that makes me that way. I want to be loving, selfless. Help me, Lord, to react in love instead of defense. I fear being broken. I fear not being loved. I fear making a fool of myself. Help me to let go of my ego. Let it be replaced with your loving presence. Help me! Help me, Bev

Mounting Limitations

Devotion

What kind of emotional baggage do you carry with you? Fear, doubt, anxiety, and confusion weigh heavily on us. I take with me the load of yesterday's problems and the worry of what tomorrow may bring which blocks the way to happiness. I am challenged to live in the glory of today, and in Jesus Christ for truth, light, and love. Christ reveals himself to us. Jesus tells us He will take our burdens and we can be free from the burdens we hold on to.

Psalm 55:22
> Cast your burden on the Lord, and He shall sustain you; He shall never permit the righteous to be moved.

God is glad to carry your burdens and give you the daily strength you need.

Let go of the burdens you carry around. You don't need to carry this by yourself. His strength is perfect and is all that I need.

Thankful for hope.

11/2005

My Jesus, for many years, I have been aware, have open to, those hidden springs of hope. These last few years have been hard on me; my children, my parents, my diminishment. But Lord, I am ever grateful for the grace of hope. Even in my despair, I know you come with that hope. Not always with the face I expect, I don't recognize your gift of hope. But, my Lord, the hope is there and when I embrace it, new life can come. It is always in the agony, the dying, the resurrection. Help me to hope. I can get so easily into my pity pot. Lord, I believe, help my unbelief.

Devotion

Theologian Emil Brunner said, "What oxygen is for the lungs; such is hope for the meaning of human life." If hope is the meaning for life and is essential, then why do I see so much despair and hopelessness? Situations happen that are just unfair. We question where is God in all of this? Why would He let such a thing happen? Our faith is easily shaken. It simply does not compute in my mind.

I Peter 5:6
> Humble yourselves, therefore, under God's mighty hand, that He may lift you up in due time.

There is a time factor to this that I am not always comfortable with. Christ asks me to trust him and wait on Him in all circumstances. He asks me to cast my cares on Him. Why? Because He cares for me, He loves me, He doesn't want me to suffer. I wonder why I hold on to so many things instead of laying them at His feet? Remembering He is here, loving me, wanting what is best for me is what keeps me hanging on.

It isn't always easy, but I can't give up, because He hasn't given

Mounting Limitations

up. I am challenged to continue living in His presence and do all things with a joyful heart, especially when I am hurting and don't understand. I only see a portion of what is happening and I call it unjust and unfair. There is much more that I cannot comprehend that God knows. He loves me too much to let me suffer alone. God sees my heart and knows when I choose to be obedient to Him. I am comforted in knowing in my time of sorrow and despair when things seem hopeless, Christ is with me and still brings joy in these tough times. In order to make sense as to why I can still have joy in troubled times, I believe and live the following verse in the poem "Not Knowing" written by Mary Gardiner Brainard—"I would rather walk in the dark with God, than walk alone in the light."

A new awareness of not being who she used to be:

12/10/2005
Psalm 80:18-19

> Then we will not turn away from you; revive us, and we will call on your name. Restore us, Lord God Almighty; make your face shine on us, that we may be saved.

My Jesus, I long to have the presence of mind I once had. The awareness of your presence in all. Oh, it's still present, but I feel somehow disconnected, scattered, out of focus. I long for that special intimacy I have felt. I know your presence is always there, but I feel disconnected, lost in a maze. Then fear takes over, and I can no longer think rationally. Lord, bring me peace. Love, Bev

8/20/2006
John 6:57-58

> Just as the living Father sent me and I live because of the Father, so the one who feeds on me will live because of me. This is the bread that came down from heaven. Your ancestors ate manna and died, but whoever feeds on this bread will live forever.

My Jesus, can I integrate within myself your life and your sacrifice? Only with your presence to me. Your grace is all I need. Yet as I say this, I am resistant. I do not like to hurt in any form. Yet, Lord, your example is through pain and resurrection. In a way I feel I am going through that cycle. Walking in your footsteps in the sense that I am being discriminated against because of things I cannot control. But, I see no other way. Also as you indicate through your life, there will be pain. There must be a death, a giving up control to the Father. A surrender to His will. I resist because I fear. What will become of me? What will others think? I fear the loss of community. I need people around. I need to be doing something. I do not want to be a burden on anyone. Help me accept whatever is my journey. Please, my Jesus, keep me always present to you, your love. Amen.

1/28/2006

"Failures are opportunities to improve. You can't get better until you see what's wrong."
My Jesus, I have spent a lot of energy on denying that something is wrong (health wise, memory wise). It is accepting the possibility and taking steps for help that new life has emerged. New life in quietness of soul, new life in knowing what a day is. It is the calm within that has taken over the inner panic. Lord,

Mounting Limitations

I truly want to have peace with those that have caused me pain and stress. I want to be able to forgive and let go of the anger and disappointment, the hurt. Teach me to love as you love. Amen.

2/1/2006
2 Samuel 24:10-17

>David was conscience-stricken after he had counted the fighting men, and he said to the Lord, "I have sinned greatly in what I have done. Now, Lord, I beg you, take away the guilt of your servant. I have done a very foolish thing." Before David got up the next morning, the word of the Lord had come to Gad the prophet, David's seer: "Go and tell David, 'This is what the Lord says: I am giving you three options. Choose one of them for me to carry out against you.'" So Gad went to David and said to him, "Shall there come on you three years of famine in your land? Or three months of fleeing from your enemies while they pursue you? Or three days of plague in your land? Now then, think it over and decide how I should answer the one who sent me." David said to Gad, "I am in deep distress. Let us fall into the hands of the Lord, for his mercy is great; but do not let me fall into human hands."
>
>So the Lord sent a plague on Israel from that morning until the end of the time designated, and seventy thousand of the people from Dan to Beersheba died. When the angel stretched out his hand to destroy Jerusalem, the Lord relented concerning the disaster and said to the angel who was afflicting the people, "Enough! Withdraw your hand." The angel of the Lord was then at the threshing floor of Araunah the Jebusite.

> When David saw the angel who was striking down the people, he said to the Lord, "I have sinned; I, the shepherd, have done wrong. These are but sheep. What have they done? Let your hand fall on me and my family."

My Jesus, two things strike me. The "pestilence" which David chose from his choices. For me this sounds like an extended time of unrest within— discord among the people. It makes me reflect on those things in my life that are pitfalls, things that happen that distract from God. Like when things are going well, and something happens to break my peace. How it rattles me, breaks "my" peace, "my" plans. There have been times in the last few years that I have felt the pestilence. My world never seems calm for very long. Always a cog to divert. My Jesus, you have been my mainstay. You are my rock. Thank you, thank you. Lord, help me to recognize you within the pestilence, the chaos. Amen.

3/16/2008

The story of the Prodigal Son
I know today my parents are completely dependent on me. I know the lessons I am being taught in love and forgiveness. You cannot turn my back on a lost sheep; lost in the sense of lost memory, lost physical and mental capacity. Jesus speaks of embracing the little children, elderly, especially those with dementia, are like little children. At least their needs are those of children; to be loved and cared for having a safe place to be who they are at the moment. My Jesus, as the father embraced and forgave the wayward son, I ask for forgiveness of my sinfulness, and I ask for the presence of your spirit in all my encounters and within my heart. Lord, I want to be like you, loving and forgiving. Love, Beverly

Mounting Limitations

8/23/2006
Psalm 23:6

> Surely your goodness and love will follow me all the days of my life, and I will dwell in the house of the Lord forever.

My Jesus, this is such a comforting statement. It reassures me of your presence here and now and for the future. I know how desperately I need your presence in the "now." I cannot depend on myself, sometimes I do not know me. Help me Lord to always remember that you are always with me. Amen.

Devotion

We've been brought up to believe, "You can do anything." Just believing that you can do something doesn't mean you really can, at least through your own strength.

Proverbs 3:5-6

> Trust in the LORD with all your heart and lean not on your own understanding; in all your ways acknowledge him, and he will make your paths straight.

I don't know about you, but I tend to lean on my own understanding. I depend on my own strength most of the time. Mom probably did too, but is now realizing she can't rely on herself any longer. This reminds me that there are times when no matter how much I try; I cannot do it on my own.

There are times in life that the only way I will be able to go on is to trust in Christ for His strength to get me through. I won't ever understand why there is a disease that leaves the outline of a person, but slowly takes away everything that is on the inside. I can't imagine how painful it is to live through this, (and I realize one day I might) but I do know the pain in watching the struggle and not being able to do anything about it. I trust without understanding, and I know without a doubt that my God is present with me and still with Mom every single day.

9/2006

My Jesus, I am certainly in a place of indifference, do I stay or do I go? I know these past few years have taken a toll on me, mentally and emotionally. I am ready for a respite. My own diminishment weighs heavy on me. Fear sets in. Help me Lord to understand what you are calling me to and how to negotiate it well. Be my guide!
Beverly

Devotion

Have you ever gotten stuck in a spiritual rut, not knowing what to do next? You know what you should do but can't seem to make yourself get up and do it. Ignatius of Loyola wrote, "In times of dryness and desolation we must be patient . . . putting our trust in the goodness of God. We must animate ourselves by the thought that God is always with us, that He only allows

Mounting Limitations

this trial for our greater good, and that we have not necessarily lost His grace because we have lost the taste and feeling of it."

We are not alone in feeling this emptiness. There was an occasion recorded in Numbers 11:15 when Moses shouted at God: "If this is how you are going to treat me, please go ahead and kill me—if I have found favor in your eyes—and do not let me face my own ruin." During these times, I have to intentionally choose faith over understanding.

9/2006
I Cor. 13:12-13

> For now we see only a reflection as in a mirror; then we shall see face to face. Now I know in part; then I shall know fully, even as I am fully known.
>
> And now these three remain: faith, hope and love. But the greatest of these is love.

My Jesus, self-knowledge comes only through the presence and love of God. There are times, my Jesus, I would rather not know myself. I want to live in my illusions. It is easier. However, peace does not come in illusions. It is the acceptance of what is that brings peace. What is, is that I am aging. I am having moments of forgetfulness that are very frightening. In my efforts to "run away" I am losing myself.

There are times I do not know who I am. Fleeting moments, but fearful moments. This I do know, you will take care of me, love me even when I am unloving. I know I am an alarmist Lord, temper me. Give me surrender to your will and trust in your eternal and perfect love.

Devotion

Don't we all have illusions of who we are and how we want things to be? Do we live in a world that is an illusion that will eventually lead to disillusion because we haven't been honest with ourselves? Sometimes I deny the problem by saying, "All is good," without facing the problem.

Other times I face the problem head-on, but dwell in that place not moving forward. What a destructive place that is, to be paralyzed in my disappointment/disillusionment. This is when my heart becomes hard, and I become bitter. I must be careful that my disillusions don't go too far and blame God for the hardships I face.

God does allow things to happen, but He is not the creator of evil and suffering. He is never out to get me. Not only does God hear our cries but cries with us. When we hurt, he hurts all the more because of how much he loves us. Recognizing the limits of my perspective is essential. Christ truly loves us in a way we can't comprehend. I let him down and turn my back on him often. It's easy to blame God for circumstances I face. His unconditional love for me when I am unlovable can be too incredible to believe, especially when things don't match my way of thinking.

I Corinthians 13:12
> Now we see things imperfectly, like puzzling reflections in a mirror, but then we will see everything with perfect clarity. All that I know now is partial and incomplete, but then I will know everything

Mounting Limitations

completely, just as God now knows me completely.

It was some time during this year she started missing appointments and forgetting small things. Her work was suffering. She set up appointments at home, but she wouldn't be there. Although she was embarrased, she always had an excuse to hide her forgetfulness. All the while, she was tormented inside wondering if, when, and how this would get worse. She built up walls to protect herself, but still tried to be kind and loving like Christ. The conflict inside created moodiness and inconsistent behaviors.

10/2006
Philippians 3:8
> What is more, I consider everything a loss because of the surpassing worth of knowing Christ Jesus my Lord, for whose sake I have lost all things. I consider them garbage, that I may gain Christ.

As I struggle with this memory thing, I have come to know in a very concrete way that dependence on you is essential. Fear of the future overwhelms me at times. Yet you give me the hope to walk on. To trust in your will for me and the grace to discern my will from yours; not an easy task. Decisions are not easy for me. Fear is a great obstacle for me. The desire to trust is sometimes overrun by fear and rejection of the reality of things. Teach me surrender and trust. Amen.

Devotion

Surrender what? Surrender God's healing? Surrender to the

demise of this disease? It's not giving up or giving into the disease, but surrender to fighting against the disease, surrender into acceptance of what will be.

Surrender in pretending things are OK. Surrender is accepting things are as they are now and being open to changes that will happen.

Trust always goes along with surrender. Surrender is scary. Trusting in knowing that whatever happens, God will take care of you. Healing can occur in many ways; emotions, relationships, and spiritual healing.

Surrender may mean to slow down, being honest about your thoughts and feelings and letting go to let God deal with these issues. It is when I surrender that I can fulfill the highest purpose for my life at that moment and have the most potential. Mom learns that when you get hurt, get rejected, get misrepresented when overlooked, there is only one way to respond, that is to keep on living.

Respond with trust and surrender to God. She often thanks God for the realization and to learn from it. What strength this woman had to put so much faith and hope in God when she could not see it. Faith is believing when we do not see. (Hebrew 11:1)

2006
2 Corinthians 6:2

> For he says, 'In the time of my favor I heard you, and in the day of salvation I helped you.' I tell you, now is the time of God's favor, now is the day of salvation.

My Jesus, I long for this day of salvation. A day that I can feel

Mounting Limitations

myself whole again body and mind working in tandem, being at peace. I long to trust in what I'm saying and thinking as what is proper, valid, on target. It is so lonely to live in this place of not knowing, not remembering. I am forced to live in the moment, but a moment means not always having a history bank from which to draw. There are times for me that I am like the man in "Ground Hog Day." I have to begin a new each time. I need to be reminded over and over again.

2006

My Jesus, it is so frightening. Can you please help me? I'm not functioning well in society. I have the sincerest desire to, but my memory won't cooperate. I need healing. I need acceptance. HELP Amen.

2006

My Jesus, your love and presence is all I need. Help me to continually attach myself to you. You, Lord, know the pain of rejection, the fear of loneliness of not knowing. The fear of not being able to do for yourself. The humility to surrender to what is and to trust in the Father's love. Brother Jesus, teach me to trust, to surrender, to love as you love. Please show me how and walk with me through it. Love, Bev

Devotion

Mom longs for the day of salvation that comes through his mercy directly from grace. We do not know the day or hour.

An Introspective Journey

There's no way of knowing when that day will come. We have to be prepared. We will die and have to stand before the Father and the Righteousness of His Son. Mom is right with God. She has lived a lifestyle of repentance and surrender. She is ready to surrender her past and live in the moment. She knows she is being attacked in her mind. She knows the feelings of rejection. She recognizes that Jesus suffered pain and rejection too. She can submit herself to God knowing Jesus was able to surrender and submit to His father also.

11/14/2006
2 Timothy 2:13

> If we are faithless, he remains faithful, for he cannot disown himself.

This speaks to me in a powerful way. It is overwhelming to hear the depths that each individual "me" is rooted in the heart of God. It humbles me. How unworthy I am to receive such love and presence of the Holy. My Lord and my God, I'm so grateful for that love. In this time of my life where I get confused, lose focus, get lost, to be assured in your presence, you care and love is so comforting. Thank you, thank you. Beverly

Devotion

What a remarkable thought that even when my faith is weak, He remains faithful. God's grace is not based on my faith, but He is faithful. It doesn't depend on me. I am not entirely

Mounting Limitations

faithful in doing what I should. His character says that when He makes a promise, He will keep it. His love has proved it. He endured everything to save me, a sinner. The God of the universe delights in me. How do I treat Jesus in my daily life? Do I take His love for granted?

2006

I am in flux between what I want and what you want for me. Help me, Jesus, to recognize your voice in the midst of the busyness of my life. I long for inner peace. I used to think that I was sure of everything, I knew the task, but I am not sure anymore. I continue to struggle within myself. These last 2 days have been good. Community with my cousins, lunch with friends today. These gifts I thank you for. I feel truly blessed today. I know that this will not be for always. Spirit of Jesus heal me of this negativity and distrust. I believe you can heal me, give me peace and give me a Spirit of hope, trust, and love for all things and all people. Distrust seems to be my biggest obstacle. Infuse me with trust in you and trust in others. Heal me of the pain inside. Show me how to truly love. Amen.

She worked so hard at remembering. She wrote everything down. She had sticky notes to remind her of things, on the fridge, wall, wherever she thought it could help her. She adopted strategies to organize and reorganize. Her journal writings were scattered. She wrote in different notebooks during the same time frame. Sometimes she wrote from the back of the notebook instead of where she had left off.

It was also growing nearer for Dad's retirement. From the

perspective of their children, we wondered if Dad was retiring because he knew she needed more help with her daily life. Did he retire at this time to take care of her?

Some of her prayers are answered because they began going on more trips together. Their days were not stagnant as she once feared. Dad has great comfort that they had this time together, the time of putting it off to another day had past and that day and time had come.

1/19/2007

My Jesus, I am in a quandary. I want to have friends to do things with, couples, but Paul seems almost anti-social. I'm saddened, and I'm longing for some excitement, some activity to be a part of that we could do together. I fear his retirement. What will be expected of me? Is all we will do be around the house? I need interaction with others. Help me Jesus to motivate him into losing weight so that he can exercise properly and consistently, and me too. It was very lonely yesterday evening. We hardly spoke to each other, just watched TV. Please my Jesus, help us both as we move into this next phase of our lives, retirement. Give me grace of patience and insight to help him to see his possibilities.

It was during this time Mom and Dad starting going on a lot of vacations. Most often with friends on cruises. I believe watching her mother and father deal with their illnesses gave her a nudge to live life to the fullest and enjoy life while they could.

I had the shock of my life one evening. I received a call from Mom when she and Dad were on a trip in Puerto Rico. She told me she was lost and needed me to come and get her. I kept thinking, "Do they speak English over there? Who do I call?"

Mounting Limitations

My husband immediately tried calling Dad on his cell phone with no luck while I tried to get Mom to explain where she was. She just kept telling me she was in the same place where I left her a few minutes before.

She said, "Paul and the others were here just now, and when I turned around, they were gone. They have all left me. I don't know where they all went."

The phone connection was poor, and the call kept getting dropped. I kept calling her back until she stopped answering the phone. A panic like I've never felt before overcame me. What do I do? Who do I call? How can we find Mom who is lost somewhere in Puerto Rico? We kept calling both her phone and Dad's phone. A few hours later, Dad picked up as if there was nothing wrong. He said they were fine and got off the phone without acknowledging what had occurred. Talk about being left to hang there. I knew they were safe and that is all that mattered.

What actually happened may always be a mystery. I got two stories from Dad. One is that they signed up for an excursion that required her to wear a bathing suit. The excursion took them out to a bioluminescent lagoon at nightfall where the water glows fluorescent with every movement and splash due to the microscopic plankton that live in the waters. Despite reminders, she had not worn her bathing suit. She was not allowed on the excursion and agreed to sit and wait until the others returned. The other story is that when time came for her to get on the boat, she refused. No one could convince her to get in. Neither Dad or her friends cruising with her had a clue her memory was so poor. They did not understand her actions. Dad experienced many similar incidences and dealt with them the best he could. He had no one to talk to but held it all inside simply trying to love his wife.

Devotion

We are not meant to carry your burdens alone. Gal. 6: 1-10 explains how we need each other, being careful not to think too highly of ourselves or comparing ourselves with each other. We need our spiritual family. We all need to have someone we can call on when life is tough. I need someone who will hold me accountable, even if it is difficult. Someone I can trust, to pray with me, and someone I can enjoy the presence of God with. My spiritual family can and does help me carry my burdens. There have been numerous times I was under heavy stress and I knew I had someone lifting me in prayer.

I feel His presence more clearly in the stressful times than I do when things are going well for me. Times I when I know I can't handle things on my own, but supernaturally am given the strength, wisdom, courage, and patience I need at the moment. When dealing with the ongoings of this disease, we often hide from others our struggles and trials. There are so many other just like you, others that can offer you support in this time. Ask God to bring someone in your life that can help you during this struggle. The unbearable will become bearable when you let others bear the burden with you.

My immediate family started to try to include Mom and Dad in more of our vacations and trips knowing our time was limited. We mostly did things that would let them relax and enjoy God's beautiful world. We went to see waterfalls and mountains, things that were calm and peaceful; things that did not require

Mounting Limitations

anything but being in the present. Often times as we drove in the countryside, Mom would rattle on and on about the area, about events that happened at this place as she was growing up there. She'd point out places where something significant had happened when she was younger. It sounded so believable. I'm sure those event happened, but we were not anywhere near the area she grew up. That didn't matter. She was sharing the feelings this place took her to. Instead of arguing with her on the logistics of where she was, it was easier to enjoy hearing of the stories from her past.

We can't dwell on specifics that this disease takes away, but for as long as we can, we can cherish the moments we still have with her. We can help her keep her dignity, respect her as a person, and love the person we know she is inside.

Chapter 6

NO MORE HIDING FROM REALITY

She fears unacceptable behavior creeping into her life.

1/27/2007

My Jesus, help me to be loving and kind. Give me the strength I need to be that loving person you created. I long for inner peace. I want to be productive. But, Jesus, I can't always do these things. My health is a limitation. Sometimes I do not know who I am. I know my name, etc. What I do not know is why I do and say some things. I fear that my inability to discern, I will say and do unacceptable behavior. Lord, help me to be kind and loving. Help me also to find some means of active (physical) and mental exercise that will sustain a productive life.

A few years later, her fears of having unacceptable behavior and saying things became a reality. People noticed, but didn't understand. No one was aware of the internal struggle and the impact this disease was having on her. At times she was just downright mean and hateful. Many days it came out of nowhere, the anger and accusations that were off based and irrational. I don't think anyone realized that Mom comprehended what was happening to her. On some levels, she did, and in other ways, she did not.

Eventually, we learned there was no winning the argument. One weekend the whole family was together, my brother and my family stayed at Mom and Dad's house. It was early in the morning, and not everyone was up yet. I was helping Mom in the kitchen when she walked up to me with fire in her eyes. She vigorously shook her finger at me and with a firm, serious look, lit into me.

"I don't like the way you are treating me! You do what you want and what is convenient for you. You only care about yourself. You are only out for what you can get out of me. You don't care about me, and I don't even like going to visit you. It's so hard to be with you!"

The anger in which she spoke tore into my heart. My mind told me I didn't deserve this thrashing. I wanted to defend myself from these accusations that came from out of the blue, and ask, "What are you talking about?" I knew if I had asked, she couldn't give me anything specific. She only knew how she felt.

So often she spoke gently to me and always talked about how much she enjoyed coming to see me and spend time with me. This was so contrary to everything I thought or everything she normally said. My head knew what she was saying was irrational, but she was so sure of herself and believed she was being wronged. Her thoughts of my actions were very painful to her. She had to "defend" herself and let me know how she was being treated was not OK.

I fought back the tears of hurt, not just from the hateful words that had been spoken to me, but hurt that she believed them, that her mind was doing this to her. My heart ached knowing how she was hurting and knowing there was nothing I could do to help her. There were no words to say that could take this away. Mom was tormented by this disease.

I wasn't the only one who was treated so harshly. All of us kids, as well as Dad, had our turn. The thing is, I could walk away from her and a few minutes later, I am still hurting, angry, and upset, but she has no recollection of the events that had just occurred.

We didn't want to believe it was true. Denial is having one eye closed to reality. But denial, at least for both Mom and Dad, in their own way was the only way to make sense and have some kind of normalcy in a world that was turned upside down. It was their coping mechanism. No longer could we pretend these things weren't happening. No matter how hard we pretended these problems didn't exist, it could not cure Alzheimer's. This disease wouldn't go away.

The load was mostly on Dad. The love he had for his wife would be tested in a way he never could imagine. He tenderly guided her around everywhere and did his best to cover up her mistakes.

2/10/2007

My Jesus, it is true I do not always accept that I am loved and forgiven. I know in my heart I am loved, but my head continues to question myself. For some reason, I equate being loved with words and actions from others. I so often, depend on acceptance from others to evaluate my worth. I have especially lately, with the memory deficit, felt less than whole. Help me Lord to find a resting place. Give me people who can accept the not so perfect, and can love me. Help me my Jesus to be at peace. I have a great deal of fear. Amen.

Ultimately, her behaviors exacerbated. She could no longer

remember how to do so many things. Her daily life skills were diminishing. Her cooking is limited. She didn't cook at all if it were just her and Dad, but when company came, she felt she had to prepare meals.

This is what cooking was like for Mom. Being in Louisiana, rice was almost always part of a big dinner. She'd pour a random amount of uncooked rice in the pot. She then put in a random amount of water. The pot was put on the stove. Sometimes the stove was on, sometimes not. I'd have to wait until she walked out of the room or turned her back and adjust the amount of water and adjust the stove temperature correctly. Catching me adjust what she had just done was not acceptable, and boy did I hear it if I got caught. She might walk out of the room for perhaps five minutes and return. She would look at the pot of rice, put the lid on and turn it off. Again, when she wasn't looking, I'd turn it back on to cook. Sometimes she would put the stove on high, and the water would cook down, and the food would burn. Routinely she would overcook or under-cook her food. It was exhausting watching what she did, then follow behind her to fix it without her knowledge. She was always on the move and you couldn't take your eyes off of her for a minute.

The fire alarm went off more than we'd like to remember because she had left something on the stove and forgot about it. One Sunday morning, Mom and Dad went to church when she left something on the stove. The fire department showed up about the same time they did after Mass. I came by a bit later to see all the doors and windows open letting out the smoke. I asked Dad to unplug the electric stove to avoid any danger. He never did. I'm not sure he ever realized how dangerous it was. He always thought he'd be there and be able to avoid any accidents. I thank God that no damage was ever done, and no one was ever hurt.

She would always make a plate of food for Dad. Her

combinations were strange, but whatever she put in front of Dad, he ate it as inedible or unappealing as it may be. I felt so sorry for him. She would be offended and become upset if he changed anything about what she fixed him. She was loving and serving her husband the best way she knew how.

Mom couldn't remember things that had happened just minutes before. She would look around her and assume she had done whatever she saw. She took credit for anything and everything around her. She couldn't really cook any longer, but believed she could. We would all pitch in, bring food over, and set a beautiful table.

I recall one holiday, after setting up the table for her, she came by and admired the table decorations "she had done" and even took pictures. She would be so proud of the beautiful meal "she had prepared."

I can hear her now declaring, "This was really good. I guess I still can cook. I'm proud of myself."

This would include the fresh cake that we bought at the bakery. She also craved reinforcement of gratitude from others. She longed to hear from others how wonderful she had made things because in her mind she was doing everything she knew how to make things special for her company. If no one recognized her effort, she would become agitated. She shared with Dad that she felt that no one cared about her feelings and the hard work she put into it. She wanted to feel appreciated. It was as if her self-value depended on what others thought.

Dad would often whisper to family members reminding us to make sure to make a big deal at how nice she prepared things and how much we appreciated her regardless if she had done anything or not.

2/11/2007

No more Hiding from Reality

My Jesus, I continue to re-read about acceptance. That God can listen and even hear what is left unsaid and still really love me and accept me. God is the deepest ground of my living. I continually want proof of love; need proof that I am loved and accepted. It has become particularly important to know I am loved because of the confusion that has come into my head. I so long for my old life of energy and excitement; always new and exciting. My life seems so dull. There is no joy. God lives in the ever present NOW! The whole of time is condensed in this one moment — ever present moment. God's time is condensed in this every present now! Lord, help me to remember this always.

Devotion

How often do we get so caught up in the details of everyday life that we just don't have time to seize the moment? We've got deadlines and commitments, problems and priorities, distractions and obstacles, and though we really want more fulfillment from each day, it just doesn't seem to be within our grasp.

"Jesus said, 'No procrastination. No backward looks. You can't put God's kingdom off till tomorrow. Seize the day.'" (Luke 9:62 MSG) Am I putting off doing something today because it is not part of my deadlines of what I plan to accomplish? Are there things I need to do to be present to Christ today? What do I need to be doing to let others know about God's love, acceptance, and forgiveness? Am I missing the moment because I'm too caught up in reaching for the future? Am I too caught up in myself?

An Introspective Journey

Friends are becoming increasingly concerned and start asking questions. It is difficult to share with her friends and extended family when we are told so little of what was going on. But the decline was evident. We continued pretending to the outside world that things were fine when inwardly knew something was going terribly wrong.

We no longer could trust the accuracy of information Mom gave. Usually, parts of what she said were true, but the details were made up. It's so strange because she believed what she said. In the beginning, Dad would correct her, but after she would argue that she knew what she said was right, he eventually gave up and let her talk.

Most of the conversations were superficial. If asked, "Mom, what have you been doing today?" She would come up with the craziest stuff to say. She'd give a list of where they went and who they had visited that day. Dad never corrected her but would shake his head "no" behind her back to let us know it wasn't true. Usually they had just been home watching television. Many times she thought she had just returned from a trip and she would say, "It will be so nice to sleep in my own bed tonight."

When we needed accurate information, we needed to ask Dad. Mom's discernment in the moment was sharp, and she picked up on this trend. If we directed our questions to him, looked at him and not at her, her feelings were hurt. She became paranoid about what we might be saying to Dad if she couldn't hear the conversation. All phone calls were immediately put on speaker phone. Dad made the request that when we call on their cell phones, to always call Mom's cell first; not his. If we called Dad and not her, she thought we were ignoring her. Her paranoia was growing, which included her family that loves her. Still through all of her limitations, she continued writing about giving thanks for what she can still do and accomplish.

No more Hiding from Reality

8/2007
Psalm 138: 3

> On the day I cried out, you answered me. You encouraged me with inner strength.

My Jesus, you have been wonderful in helping me negotiate this health problem. This loss of memory, my slow response. However, I still do not know what it is you want from me in this experience. I am so filled with the thoughts of what from me. I long to live life more fully. Just when I am ready and able to be completely vulnerable. I am not sure exactly who I am. I am not who I was or, at times, I am not someone I even recognize. I long to be who you expect and hope for me. Teach me to love, teach me selflessness, teach me humility, teach me to love. Bring me peace.

9/29/2007

Lord, if at all possible, let this ugliness inside of me that spills over onto others, heal the person that has triggered my disease. I know it's a judgment, but I think he is also in need of healing. Give me the grace to love and forgive. I can only do this with your help, your love and your grace. Give me too, Lord, the words of reconciliation with those who seem to have been hurt by my actions.

10/6/2007
Psalm 69:33-37

> The Lord hears the needy and does not despise his captive people. Let heaven and earth praise him, the seas and all that move in them, for God will save Zion and rebuild the cities of Judah. Then people will settle there and possess it; the children of his

servants will inherit it, and those who love his name will dwell there.

My Jesus, I am in bondage. My loss of memory, the paranoia that seems to be creeping into my perceptions when I feel attacked. My defense mechanisms react inappropriately. Lord, I want to be kind and I want to be liked and appreciated. Help me Lord to navigate this time in my life with kindness and love.

10/14/2007
Matthew 8 1-4

> When Jesus came down from the mountainside, large crowds followed him. A man with leprosy came and knelt before him and said, "Lord, if you are willing, you can make me clean." Jesus reached out his hand and touched the man. "I am willing," he said. "Be clean!" Immediately he was cleansed of his leprosy. Then Jesus said to him, "See that you don't tell anyone. But go, show yourself to the priest and offer the gift Moses commanded, as a testimony to them."

My Jesus, today's gospel on healing the leper calls me to examine my life. Am I the leper or am I those who shun and disregard and avoid the leper? I identify today with the leper since my memory has been failing and my perceptions of things have been distorted. People who were friends have distanced themselves from me. In some ways I am a leper. Lord, help me to trust in your love from; that I am safe in your love. I want to be productive. I want to be useful. I want to be "in the world"; enjoying it. Teach me and lead me through this new way of being. Lead me to those places of productivity. Help Paul to find those places too. Help me. I want to be doing and being.

No more Hiding from Reality

10/15/2007

Lord, there are times I am not sure of who I am. The me that tries to erupt is not an acceptable personality. I want to be loved for myself. I believe that you love me for myself, but I don't always know who I am. Teach me to love as you love- especially myself. Amen.

10/29/2007

My Jesus, I long for the closeness we have had in the past. My world, my life situations have robbed me of my peace. Granted, I have in a sense let it happen. So many times in the past several years I have felt the loss of control in my own life.... fear and disappointment of myself and of others. I have felt so totally isolated from companionship with others. Why is it Lord that I need so much affirmation? Help me to trust in your love for me just as I am so that I can have the courage to step out to the unfamiliar, so I can love with complete trust. Help me Jesus!

11/14/2007

Wisdom 6:1-11
   "Therefore, desire my word..."

My Jesus, I desire your word; however, I easily forget my intent to listen to act on your word. The call to love is waylaid by my need to be "right," "accepted by others," "my perceptions of others," "my" desire to do good and the good is invalidated by my actions. Actions the fuel for the ego. I really hate myself in these times. I know you love me, yet how can you love such as me? I desire to love completely. You and those I am closest to. I do love. I just

An Introspective Journey

can't seem to get beyond my own ego. I want to think first of others, then myself. I want the grace of self-surrender to your will and surrender to your spirit moving in me. Heal me Lord. Give me the gift of kindness, compassion and self-surrender. I want to be your servant. I want others to see you in me. Amen.

> "The Holy Spirit is present within each moment and particle of existence."
>
> Orson Pratt

12/3/2007

My Jesus, I long to be the person you have called me to be. This may be who you want, but you and I know I can't be finished yet! I long to be a loving person, a giving person, a kind person.... coming to the realization of my many faults I want to change. Keep the good and transform that which needs healing and redirection. All the pains of rejection keep haunting me. It's my unhealthy defenses that keep popping up. Lord, I want to be selfless, to be for others, to be a face of your presence in my home and family and in my world. Please heal me of the fear of rejection. The fear of losing my mind. Heal me Lord of the fear that causes my outbursts of "whatever." I am so afraid of rejection, of embarrassing myself and others in a "demented" moment. Direct me to the activities and interactions with others that honor you, my Lord and that will always respect my personal dignity and those of others. Show me your face in all I encounter. Heal me of that jealousy that has been popping up. Please guide me, let me speak your words and act in ways that give you honor. Help me!
Bev.

12/25/2007

No more Hiding from Reality

My Jesus, I long to have a joyful heart that I would have the gift of positive thinking, that I could see the best instead of the negative in each encounter and thought. The angels rejoice, and the world was given hope. It is hope that I wish I had. With hope, I could first see the positive, with hope I could be free of negativity. It is hope, Lord, that you came to bring to the world on that first Christmas along with trust in the Father's will. I long to be an optimist, to trust in the path you put before me. Give the grace to be a face love and joy with my children and grandchildren this week. Thank you for Paul, so patient with my mood swings, so loving. I want to be like me again. My Jesus, I do not want to be this mean person that keeps me trying to take over. Help me Jesus on this first day of hope, of peace, and of love. Bev

12/13/2007

My Jesus, I want to do "good" but many times I don't move into action quick enough. By the time I act the need no longer exists. It's as though I'm in a dead space, half present, half absent. Give me the grace to be present and aware of others' needs and the grace to act on it. Give me your love and your grace, that is enough for me. Love, Bev.

1/7/2008

I John 4:11-12

> Dear friends, since God so loved us, we also ought to love one another. No one has ever seen God; but if we love one another, God lives in us and his love is made complete in us.

My Jesus, I want to so desperately to be loved, yet, I'm not sure

An Introspective Journey

I am a lovable person. I long to be loveable, to be well thought of, but I do things so spontaneously that is not loving. My Jesus, heal me, expel this demon that lives within me. Give me stronger armor to protect my fragile ego. I beg you Lord for this grace. As you said that last night "take this cup away." I ask to take this meanness in me away, this distrust, this need to be liked. Since I'm asking for, perhaps the impossible thing or things I need to deal with, I ask your will be done. And, if the answer is no, give me your heart so that I can cope with whatever the outcome is.

1/10/2008
Mark 6: 45-52

Jesus Walks on the Water

"Immediately Jesus made his disciples get into the boat and go on ahead of him to Bethsaida, while he dismissed the crowd. After leaving them, he went up on a mountainside to pray.

Later that night, the boat was in the middle of the lake, and he was alone on land. He saw the disciples straining at the oars, because the wind was against them. Shortly before dawn he went out to them, walking on the lake. He was about to pass by them, but when they saw him walking on the lake, they thought he was a ghost. They cried out, because they all saw him and were terrified.

Immediately he spoke to them and said, "Take courage! It is I. Don't be afraid." Then he climbed into the boat with them, and the wind died down. They were completely amazed, for they had not understood about the loaves; their hearts were hardened.

My Jesus, in my head I know you are there in my storms,

No more Hiding from Reality

but in the turmoil of the storm, I forget to reach out. I become engulfed in my own struggle, forget you are there just waiting or my recognition of your presence. I ask for the grace to recognize you in my storms (which are many). Help me not blow things out of proportions and to know that I am not the center of the universe. I could use a clear and focused mind. Just give me the grace of trust. Love. Amen.

Devotion

In times of turmoil in the storm, I also forget to recognize Christ's presence in the situation, or even think he may have a hidden plan for me in this place. I think of Corrie Ten Boon from her book *The Hiding Place* as she describes how God worked in prison camp she was imprisoned in during World War II for hiding Jews. Their straw-bed platforms swarmed with fleas. It was her sister, Betsie that said "Rejoice always, pray constantly, give thanks in all circumstances; for this is the will of God in Christ Jesus." That's it, Corrie! That's His answer. "Give thanks in all circumstances!" (I Thessalonians 5:18) *That's what we can do. We can start right now to thank God for every single thing about this new barracks!'*

These ladies began giving thanks to God for all circumstances knowing this was where God had placed them. As it turned out, the fleas were a blessing from God. The nuisance of the fleas also kept out the supervisors which allowed them to hold Bible Studies in the barracks. Never give up. Times will get rough. We can't always see the good or a purpose in things. We must continue praising God in all circumstances. He understands what I cannot. My mom lives in the words she wrote in her journals;

she lives in the way she interacted with others. She lives by the example she modeled throughout her life. Do I pray that she can move on to a happier place where she can understand and dance with the Father? Of course, I do. But I wait for the LORD's timing. I wait because I know God has a plan.

2/13/2008
Psalm 51:3-4; 12-13, 18-19
 Have mercy on me.

My Jesus as read this I am comforted knowing you understand my need. I do not know at times why I behave the way that I do. What I do know is that your love me, warts and all. It is that love that I long to return. I do not know how. Where do I reach out? To whom? What do I have to give to them? "God, guide my steps and bridle me with your grace." This phrase is just what I would like for myself. I so need to know that I am loved, that I am a good person, that I have worth. I seem to have embedded in me a negative spirit, a needy spirit. I need to know I am accepted that I have worth. At this point in my life, I want people and things in my life to fulfill my need to be accepted. However, I am not sure my expectations will be fulfilled and whether they should be. Only you know what it is I need. Give me the grace to recognize you in my day. Transform my mind into a positive force within me. Be with me Lord in all that I say and do. Amen.

2/21/2008
Luke 16:19-31
 "Lazarus and the Rich Man"
 "Once there was a rich man. He was dressed in

purple cloth and fine linen. He lived an easy life every day. A man named Lazarus was placed at his gate. Lazarus was a beggar. His body was covered with sores. Even dogs came and licked his sores. All he wanted was to eat what fell from the rich man's table.

"The time came when the beggar died. The angels carried him to Abraham's side. The rich man also died and was buried. In the place of the dead, the rich man was suffering terribly. He looked up and saw Abraham far away. Lazarus was by his side. So the rich man called out, 'Father Abraham! Have pity on me! Send Lazarus to dip the tip of his finger in water. Then he can cool my tongue with it. I am in terrible pain in this fire.'

"But Abraham replied, 'Son, remember what happened in your lifetime. You received your good things. Lazarus received bad things. Now he is comforted here, and you are in terrible pain. Besides, a wide space has been placed between us and you. So those who want to go from here to you can't go. And no one can cross over from there to us.'

"The rich man answered, 'Then I beg you, father Abraham. Send Lazarus to my family. I have five brothers. Let Lazarus warn them. Then they will not come to this place of terrible suffering.' "Abraham replied, 'They have the teachings of Moses and the Prophets. Let your brothers listen to them.' " 'No, father Abraham,' he said. 'But if someone from the dead goes to them, they will turn away from their sins.' "Abraham said to him, 'They do not listen to Moses and the Prophets. So they will not be convinced even if someone rises from the dead.'"

An Introspective Journey

My Jesus, I so often behave as the rich man does. Centered on self, unaware of the needs of the poor and needy and worse than that, I am not always aware of the needs of those around me. I distance myself not because of others, but because of my fear to be taken advantaged of emotionally; or fear that I will be pitied. I long to be "normal" again. But, Lord, give me the grace and awareness to live with the qualities I am given in the here and now. I am so sensitive to the attitude "momma is losing her mind"; "Don't tell her anything."

What am I do to Lord? How do I behave with my disability and at the same time being as normal as I can be? Let me know where to go from here. Is there a remedy or do I just wait for the inevitable?

Help me, Jesus, to live with kindness and joy. Give me the grace to always feel your presence. Teach me to be kind and loving. Send the spirit of my grandmother to me; kind and gentle, accepting and forgiving, always seeing the good in all things. I long for her disposition. Free me from negativity, self-centeredness, apathy, and jealousy. Give me the grace of productivity. Help me to be useful in some way. Bring me peace, but whatever you choose to do in me or not, give me the grace of acceptance. Amen.

P.S. Thank you for giving me the ability to write and the gift of trust in you.

2/26/2008

My Jesus, over the years I have resisted or I made your way fit into my way. Yet, Lord, even when my way was not your way your Holy Spirit prodded me until, after some pain and struggle, some humiliation and soul searching, my eyes are opened. I am grateful for the journey, even the pain and disappointment has brought me new awareness and with that awareness a new appreciation of

No more Hiding from Reality

your wisdom. Each time I surrender to your will (after I struggle to fit mine into the situation). I gain more insight into myself and a greater trust in your will for me. I only wish that I could come to the awareness in the moment. But, I know the struggle is the true gift. As I struggle with aging and memory deficit give me the awareness of your presence and the ability or grace to always surrender to your will for me. Teach me unconditional love for myself and for others around me. Help me to accept the imperfections of those closest to me. Always trusting in your love for them. Amen.

Dad's life was drastically changing. He could no longer do anything on his own. He had to take her everywhere he went. When he did need to leave to run errands, he went as fast as he could. But it did not matter how long he was gone, she would call him shortly after he left and shoot accusations in his direction, "How could you leave me here all alone all day long?" "I've been waiting and waiting for hours. What have you been doing?" "Who have you been with?" Her temper would get out of hand demanding him, "Come home now!" In her mind, he was doing something he should not have been doing and taking much longer than things should.

3/5/2008
John 5:30

> By myself I can do nothing; I judge only as I hear, and my judgment is just, for I seek not to please myself but him who sent me.

My Jesus, I know that my worse sense is myself. I struggle so much with wanting "my way." In some sense I need to be in control, even though in my head I know I must let go and trust.

An Introspective Journey

Everything is not in my control. I want to be in control. This loss of memory gives me even more fear in loss of control. I am not even sure of who I am at times; not my name, but who and what I am in my life. I'm fine one minute and confused the next. People around me get irritated with me. Some have chosen to avoid me. I want to be "normal" again; at least feel accepted and respected. Even my own children have written me off as incapable, "gone." It is hard to keep the balance allowing others to think as they wish without being overwhelmed by their negativity. It is painful when conversations are always directed to their father, as though I am not present. Help me Jesus to be secure in your love for me. Give me the ability to let my hurt be an offering in some way that can benefit others. "Be with me Lord when I am in trouble." This is my prayer, that you be with me always with me and that I can recognize your face in all things. Amen.

She lost things all the time. One year, she lost a pair of gold loop earrings. She searched the house high and low for them. At Christmas time, I bought her a new pair. I was so proud to be able to get her something she wanted and needed. When she opened her gift I said, "those are to replace the ones you lost."

Dad shot me a look that let me know real quick I had said something wrong. She could not accept that she would lose things. Dad often had to cover for her, buy replacements of what she lost. I found four hairdryers in her house when I cleaned it up.

It was the strangest thing the way her house became like the Bermuda Triangle. I would be there, enjoying myself, turn around and realize my purse, hat, scarf, whatever would be missing. No one could figure out where it had disappeared to. We would search the house without her knowledge and typically find the item in another room, in a closet, or in a drawer. She moved things to clean up, never realizing she was taking other people's things. She thought they belonged to her.

There were times she would be somewhere else, at church or someone's house, and believe something there was hers. So she picked it up and brought it home, after all "it was hers in the first place." Dad had to watch her very carefully and intercept when needed. Years later, when cleaning her house, we were amazed at the things we found that belonged to each of us that we didn't know where it had disappeared to. We found items in unusual places. The contents of one box we found in a bedroom included papers, a pot, clothes, picture frames, and my grandparent's marriage certificate.

Mom wants to trust, but since she can't even trust what is going on in herself, the struggle in trusting others is overwhelming.

3/7/2008

My Jesus, I have become so distrusting in other's motives toward me. I feel that I am in danger, not literally, but emotionally and spiritually. I am attacking my negative forces, yet I allow them to enter. Anger and distrust plague me. This fear of rejection plagues me always. I long for the grace of trust. Trust in others and myself. Trust that "God doesn't make trash." Trust that you are walking with me as I struggle to find my place. Teach me, Lord, to be reliant on you, on your spirit of love. I long for freedom. I long for peace... Peace within and freedom in knowing I am loved. I am a good person. I want to have friends, not just acquaintances. I guess I will forever be plagued by my past. I never learned to be generous of heart.

4/2008
John 10:7-10

Therefore, Jesus said again, "Very truly I tell you, I am the gate for the sheep. All who have come before me are thieves and robbers, but the sheep have not listened to them. I am the gate; whoever enters through me will be saved. They will come in and go out, and find pasture. The thief comes only to steal and kill and destroy; I have come that they may have life, and have it to the full.

Long have I known you are the gate. Lately, I have made that gate (you Jesus) my goal. Even now I stray. Please, my Jesus, continue to come and find me each time that I stray. And, Lord, each time give me the grace to put myself into your hands. I am struggling so much with what is causing me to be on edge, unkind. You know what I'm talking about. Give me the grace to see you in all things and in all ways. Teach me to love, my Jesus.

Devotion

I hate how I hurt the ones I love the most when I am on edge, stressed, overwhelmed. Too many times I treat strangers better than I treat my friends and family. Have you ever been in an argument at home, when the phone rings and your voice goes from yelling to a cheery, "Hello?" It happens all the time. We all do this. We all fail at love. Someone said that we hurt those we love the most. Those who know us the best are those we are most vulnerable to. It is also those that can hurt us the most.

I think about God who knows us better than anyone else. He knows everything we have done, good and bad, and those things we would be too embarrassed to mention to anyone else.

No more Hiding from Reality

Yet He lavishly loves us despite of our failures. I don't believe I truly comprehend the depth of His love for me. It's too great. Yet, every time I sin, I betray Him. I wound his heart with my thoughts and actions. I hurt the one that loves me the most, my Jesus. When I do encounter His unfailing love, I am usually moved to tears. This is the love that restores relationships and can transform anyone.

The most incredible thing about love is that the more you give love away the more it grows, regenerates, and multiplies. It is when I refuse to love, that I harbor bitterness and anger and love becomes trapped inside. What makes me strangle the one thing that brings life inside?

There is a children's book Mom used to read to us. Her eyes would always tear up as she read it because she meant every word she read. The book is *Love You Forever*, by Robert Munsch. The story starts out with a young mother rocking her baby saying, "I'll love you forever, I'll like you for always, as long as I'm living, my baby you'll be."

The story continues through the years as this child grows to adulthood, but always the mother would tell the child, "I'll love you forever, I'll like you for always, as long as I'm living, my baby you'll be."

Now as the mother becomes older and ill, her words can no longer be verbalized. Her grown adult son now holds his frail mother in his arms and lovingly speaks to her, "I'll love you forever, I'll like you for always, as long as I'm living, my mommy you'll be."

Mom may not have said those exact words to us, but certainly lived them out not just to her children, but to all those around her. We now can hold Mom's hand and say to her, "I'll love you forever,

I'll like you for always, as long as I'm living, my mommy you'll be."

4/2008
Matthew 5: 1-12

> Jesus saw the crowds. So he went up on a mountainside and sat down. His disciples came to him. Then he began to teach them.
> He said,
> "Blessed are those who are spiritually needy.
> The kingdom of heaven belongs to them.
> Blessed are those who are sad.
> They will be comforted.
> Blessed are those who are humble.
> They will be given the earth.
> Blessed are those who are hungry and thirsty for what is right.
> They will be filled.
> Blessed are those who show mercy.
> They will be shown mercy.
> Blessed are those whose hearts are pure.
> They will see God.
> Blessed are those who make peace.
> They will be called children of God.
> Blessed are those who suffer for doing what is right.
> The kingdom of heaven belongs to them.
> Blessed are you when people make fun of you and hurt you because of me. You are also blessed when they tell all kinds of evil lies about you because of me. Be joyful and glad. Your reward in heaven is great. In the same way, people hurt the prophets who lived long ago.

My Jesus, I have times of confusion. Times that I do not know

No more Hiding from Reality

what is going on, where am I going? And who and I suppose to be? I get confused; yet, I continue to walk into life. Help me my Jesus to find you in all things. To live your beatitudes, live up to your expectations for me. I struggle over and over again to stay on the path that you provide for me. Help me Lord to recognize you are in all around me. And all that is within me. To appreciate all of your wonders, all that leads me to you. Help me Jesus.

Mom is still struggling with keeping her secret from others. She especially struggles as she handles her father's funeral and extended family.

5/5/2008
"Music of the Dance"
My Jesus, I so often am deaf to your "dance," your will for me. Even when I hear the music I do not dance. I am a "watcher," an observer! I "know," but I do not act on that knowing. My Jesus, help me to hear the music and to let myself be brought into the dance, to let go of my agendas so that I can interact with the music. Give me whatever it is that is affecting my brain or whatever. Give me the strength to trust in you in all of my stress and fear of losing my mind. I do not want to be a burden on anyone. Neither do I want to be pitied. This weekend was so stressful for me, negotiating my life with others around. Help me, my Jesus to have some clarity or what is going on in my head. Teach me humility and give me a loving heart. Teach me to love unconditionally. Amen.

Devotion

I am reminded of the hymn "Lord of the Dance" by Sydney

Carter where he represents Jesus Christ as the dancing, celebrating Savior. Dancing brings joy and laughter often at a party or rejoicing over an event. Christ never wants us to forget the joy He offers to us. He wants us to be part of His life, after all that is why he came, to set us free from bondage. When I give Him my burdens, let go of my failures, accept His forgiveness, I become free and want to dance remembering the joy of the Lord is my strength. In the dance, He can lead me to the next step.

    My husband and I once took ballroom dancing. The teacher instructed me not to anticipate the next move, but to close my eyes and let my husband, the leader, guide me to the next step. When I allowed my husband lead with my eyes closed, we moved together with the music. But as soon as I starting thinking about what I was doing, I fumbled, often stepping on his toes. When I trust the true leader, my Jesus, He guides my steps into a beautiful, graceful dance. But when I take my focus off the leader, I begin to stumble. When I cling to my struggles, my will, my control then I am inhibited from dancing, hindered from receiving all that Christ desires for me. It is in the dance that I receive his mercy, grace, and inner peace.

5/27/2008

Lord, you know how I struggle with memory. Right now, help me to be calm, trusting in your guidance and care for me. Help me to relax my body, trust in your process, and to have a spirit of gratitude. Be with me Lord. Help me to have a spirit that reflects your love for me. I truly want to be the face of God to others. Amen.

No More Hiding from Reality

6/2/2008
2 Peter 1:2-11

> Grace and peace be yours in abundance through the knowledge of God and of Jesus our Lord. His divine power has given us everything we need for a godly life through our knowledge of him who called us by his own glory and goodness. Through these he has given us his very great and precious promises, so that through them you may participate in the divine nature, having escaped the corruption in the world caused by evil desires.
>
> For this very reason, make every effort to add to your faith goodness; and to goodness, knowledge; and to knowledge, self-control; and to self-control, perseverance; and to perseverance, godliness; and to godliness, mutual affection; and to mutual affection, love.
>
> For if you possess these qualities in increasing measure, they will keep you from being ineffective and unproductive in your knowledge of our Lord Jesus Christ. But whoever does not have them is nearsighted and blind, forgetting that they have been cleansed from their past sins.
>
> Therefore, my brothers and sisters, make every effort to confirm your calling and election. For if you do these things, you will never stumble, and you will receive a rich welcome into the eternal kingdom of our Lord and Savior Jesus Christ.

My Jesus, this passage is hitting me right between the eyes today. It seems it is the first time I have read it and it speaks of my reluctance to accept the pitfalls and barriers that come into my life with acceptance. I have such a resistance to change, especially change that is painful or uncertain. Change that cost me time and energy. Change that is unpleasant, anything that rocks my boat. My inability to accept that I am in "this whatever" alone and I cannot change others, that I have to accept whatever and trust in your presence. And I must love the person, not the actions. Please, my Jesus help me complete the closure of my Dad's estate with calm and peace. Give me inner peace. Amen.

Devotion

Did you know you can practice being in the presence of God? The presence of the Holy Spirit is already here. It isn't something you hope for or wish for. We don't summons it through prayer or meditation. Christ gave his Holy Spirit, but you have to accept it if you are going to recognize it around you. Become aware of this presence around you the same way you make yourself aware of the wind blowing in the trees. For me, it is being still and open to His presence. It is welcoming the Holy Spirit into my space. In dark times, it is hard to "feel" anything. As Christians, we live through faith and not feelings. There are times when being in His presence is exhilarating, overwhelming, calming and peaceful all at once. But there are times, especially in the midst of a struggle, however faint, I can know without a doubt that He is with me. That is when I experience the glory of His goodness, because I know I am not alone. He promises this in Hebrews 13:5, *"Never will I leave you; never will I forsake you."*

No more Hiding from Reality

8/27/08
Psalm 51:10

> Create in me a pure heart, O God, and renew a steadfast spirit within me.

My Jesus, for some reason my mind keeps going to the Holy Spirit. The spirit of love, the spirit of hope, the spirit of kindness. Today, 66 years ago you gave me my earthly body. I can't say that I have always treated this body and mind in a way you hoped for me. However, my Jesus, I have treasured your constant love, even when I tried to take the reins and run in the another direction. You Lord, kept watch. I am so grateful for your consistent love. I thank you for always being there for me, for putting so many wonderful people in my life to challenge me and love me. Lord, may the spirit within me be open to all reaching out in love. Give me a loving heart. Take away that meanness that keeps jumping out. Free me of negativity. Teach me to love for the sake of love, for you my Jesus, not for me. My Jesus, I put my desires my hope for freedom in your hands. Today give me a clean heart, a loving and kind heart. Amen.

Devotion

Negativity is a natural human response to things happening around us that are unpleasant. During difficult times I must search for the positive because all I can see on the surface is negative. It is a trap we have all fallen into probably more times than we care to admit. I have to stretch myself into letting Christ change my perspective. When I am in this negative attitude, I find I don't feel like doing much of anything. That is a ploy from

Satan to destroy our hope altogether. I can't let myself go deeper into the pit by allowing Satan to take away my strength, joy, and peace. John 10:10 describes Satan's goal; *"The thief cometh not, but that he may steal, and kill, and destroy: I came that they may have life, and may have [it] abundantly."*

I need to be in worship, prayer, and fellowship with others. I must spend time examining His Word and comparing it to what I am thinking and be obedient to what it tells me to do, how to live. When I am able to keep myself connected to Christ during a rough patch, Christ always shows up when I need Him most, which is usually when I am about ready to give up. I specifically ask Him to show me He is near. His actions don't always look like I expect it. And there are times when I doubt God's love rather than be comforted by it. He doesn't always take away my circumstance, but it is evident that I am not fighting this alone. Praising God in the storms of life can seem odd, and is difficult because we simply don't want to. But, that is the only way I can change my perspective, to see the positive, and begin trusting that God's got this.

9/20/08

My Jesus, I struggle so much with my loss of memory and with the recollection of information. I am not always recalling things correctly. I am frightened by this, and not sure where to go with this. Help me Lord to find peace. Do I seek a doctor or not? I am frightened to some extent, but most of all I want to know what I have to do for quality of life for me and for Paul who has to live with my behavior. My Jesus, I long for those days of knowing without a doubt. Now I am always concerned that I am mixing

No more Hiding from Reality

things up, not telling "the whole truth" or no truth at all without even knowing what I am doing. Please Jesus, help me. I long for the days of certainty, no doubts about what I say, hear or act out from. Help me Jesus to trust in your way for me. Give me and those around me the grace to love me in spite of what I say and do. But Lord, if you want to change the outcome, I am open to that. I want to stand in a place of indifference. I want to do your will. Help me Jesus to do just that. Do your will. Give me the grace to do just that. Beverly

Devotion

What wisdom I see from Mom's heart. She desperately wants to be free from this disease and asks God to "change the outcome," but is willing to accept God's will and prays for grace in acceptance of what she realizes she will live with. She is not going to get in the way of how things are to be. Nor is she going to give up on life and the potential she can still be. I am not in a place that I can say what has happened with my mom and so many others is God's will. God is infinitely good. His will for us is good also. I cannot explain why such a thing happens to someone, and I want to protest because it is not supposed to be this way. I come to grips with this because I know we are not whole here on this earth. The Lord will perfect us all in eternity. There is some comfort with this knowledge. Mom accepts what is happening and asks God to let her hurt benefit others. Her disease brought her to more reliance on Christ. I know that Christ remains with her even now when she can no longer put thoughts together to pray. Christ knows her heart. He knows my heart too. He is healing me spiritually and has also healed mom spiritually and emotionally from this disease. She is cared for in a loving environment and no longer struggles with the pain of knowing that she doesn't know. She lives in the now, no longer worrying about the past or future. In her heart, I believe she is at peace. One day, she will be healed completely and will spend eternity in the arms of Jesus and dancing in the joy of the Lord.

Chapter 7

Something's Wrong; People Notice

Conversations with Mom did become more and more difficult. When she contributed, her comments were off. She tried using cues from her surroundings to be part of the conversations. She told some stories. I don't know where the stories came from, but I don't believe she made them up completely. She believed what she was saying. It was as if she was piecing together events that had happened at different points in her life and putting them together into one mixed up story that was difficult to follow. She would repeat her story within just a few minutes of saying it or even repeat a story another person just told as if it were her idea and had not been said.

She craved interaction with others but struggled with her ability to socialize. If someone tried to correct her, she would look very hurt and not say anything else. To mention that she had already told the story would have been to add insult to injury, so everyone went along. Besides, she told stories with so much enthusiasm, we allowed her to have her moment.

A story I remember she repeated over and over was about one of her landlords when she was a young adult who had several cats. This woman would stick out her tongue and touch her nose with it like the cats did. Mom always demonstrated with her tongue stretching out to touch her nose. She repeated this same story over and over. She would laugh and laugh at the thought. I wonder if she had that story correct?

9/2008

My Jesus, my life has for many years with the mentality that if I'm good I'll be loved, but good is like beauty, in the eyes of the beholder. My idea of "good" may not be for another. Of course, there is universal good and that is you, Jesus. Being loved without attachments "if I do this or that I'll be loved." Lord, I just want to be liked, cared about. I would like a good friend, someone I could call and just talk with, but I think my crazy head has closed some doors for me. I ask for healing and for inner peace. Lord, please help me with that.
Amen.

Devotion

Why do I think everything I do has to be good and perfect or I will be condemned? I judge myself and all my faults harshly. Instead, I should strive to be faithful and should rejoice in what Christ is doing in my life. Sometimes it is baby steps, but He is always moving in my life if I let Him. No one is perfect or "good" all of the time.

Luke 5:32
> "I have not come to call the righteous, but sinners to repentance."

Something's Wrong; People Notice

I recognize that I am not good. I repent and attempt to reach perfection through Christ. I know I will never get there, but that isn't the point. It is through examining my motives, my good and bad, that I grow to rely more on Christ and begin experiencing His unconditional love. In searching the Bible, I see person after person who were not "good" and yet were used by God. My mind goes to King David.

Acts 13:22
> After removing Saul, he made David their king. God testified concerning him: 'I have found David son of Jesse, a man after my own heart; he will do everything I want him to do.'

A man after God's own heart and yet, David's life was nowhere close to being "good" all of the time. In fact, if David lived in our world today, it is likely he might be in prison. It is studying David and all these saints, I can have confidence that I'm not "good" all the time, but that doesn't stop me leading others to Christ. It is knowing His unconditional love for me personally that I can continue trying.

10/28/2008
Ephesians 4:7-16
> But to each one of us grace has been given as Christ apportioned it. This is why it says: "When he ascended on high, he took many captives and gave gifts to his people." (What does "he ascended" mean except that he also descended to the lower, earthly regions? He who descended is the very one who

ascended higher than all the heavens, in order to fill the whole universe.) So Christ himself gave the apostles, the prophets, the evangelists, the pastors and teachers, to equip his people for works of service, so that the body of Christ may be built up until we all reach unity in the faith and in the knowledge of the Son of God and become mature, attaining to the whole measure of the fullness of Christ. Then we will no longer be infants, tossed back and forth by the waves, and blown here and there by every wind of teaching and by the cunning and craftiness of people in their deceitful scheming. Instead, speaking the truth in love, we will grow to become in every respect the mature body of him who is the head, that is, Christ. From him the whole body, joined and held together by every supporting ligament, grows and builds itself up in love, as each part does its work.

My Jesus, as I read through Ephesians it strikes me how precise or rather how extensive you have prepared humanity for your presence in our world. Personality, nationality, sensitivity are all parts of our human condition you call each of us individually, taking into consideration personality, temperament, differences in processing information. This passage speaks to me about the universality of your message of love. You are saying take this information, these words of mission and love and live them with your personality your way of processing. Lord, I want to do this, but I need your grace and direction. As you know, Jesus, my mind just doesn't work as well as it once did. Please Lord, heal those parts that need repair. Show me your face in the struggle with my memory loss. My fears of abandonment, and my need to be loved,

or at least liked and respected. Give me the grace to ignore these feelings of rejection of disappointment with others. I long to be the happy go lucky person I once was. I have lost my joy. Please help me find it again.
Amen.

10/2008
Romans 5:1-11
> And hope does not put us to shame, because God's love has been poured out into our hearts through the Holy Spirit, who has been given to us. (Romans 5:5)

My Jesus, I need reconciliation within myself. To reconcile to who I am. I am a flawed person as are all humans, but my flaw is that of memory loss, of forgetfulness causing repetition in my conversations at times. I am sometimes misunderstood. I struggle so hard to be present to others. The situation yesterday spoke loudly to me. Am I being a burden on others? Is it time for me to "retire" from companions? God's love poured into my heart by the Holy Spirit. I understand that there may come a time when few will consider me as a "person" valuable. I long for clarity and presence to the moment. To make sense in my conversations. I long to be accepted just as a human being, just as I am.

Jesus, I beg you to bring clarity into my mind. Give me the grace to forgive myself and others who seem to get so bent out of shape by me. Give me, a spirit of acceptance of my family's antics. If it be your will, Lord, heal the misrepresentations of the truth. Thank you, my Jesus, for your presence in my life and thank you for Paul. Help me to always recognize the gift that he is to me. Give me the direction I need in my life to continue the journey to you. You know all the pain I feel inside of me. You know the peace I long for. My Jesus, grant me that inner peace. Amen.

11/06/2008

My Jesus, help me to trust in your way for me. Whatever you have in store for me, let me endure with dignity. I see my "person" slipping away into someone I do not know and do not want to be. I fear losing who I am and whom I know. More than anything I fear how I would behave without knowing. I fear hurting others with words that are not kind. I long to be loved (liked). Having friends gives me a sense of worthiness, in a way it validates that I am a worthwhile person. My Jesus, if it be possible, lead me to medication or whatever that can arrest this memory loss. If it be your will Lord, send me some relief. If healing of this is not your path for me, give me the grace for preservation. Show me how to live with this in dignity. I ask for forgiveness for all I have hurt in any way. Teach me to love as you love. Amen.

Devotion

Much of my self-worth comes from others. The thoughts inside me always question, "Was that good enough?" "Did that make sense?" "Do they think I'm stupid?"

Self-talk is common but can be dangerous because I see myself through the eyes of others. We all need reinforcement that we are OK. Depending on the kind of reinforcement I get will depend on my behaviors and actions. I need to keep myself from being swayed in the wind depending on others. I must set my thoughts on a foundation of truth. Mom began seeing herself through the eyes of betrayal, hurt, and rejection. It's so easy to do this. My identity is not from how others see me, but how Christ sees me. I keep my mind focused on what I know Christ says about me.

Something's Wrong; People Notice

I am a winner. Romans 8:37
I have been chosen. 1 Peter 2:9
I was made in the image of my creator. Genesis 1:27
I am designed for good works. Ephesians 2:10
I am a co-heir with Christ. Romans 8:17
I am chosen and called by God to produce fruit. John 15:16

Mom's memory comes and goes. She longs to live a normal life and thanks God for recognizing him in the everydayness of life.

11/2008

I am especially handicapped with the memory that comes and goes. I long to be secure in what I say and do, to know that I am speaking truth. It is a lonely place when others see the craziness of my mind and shun me. If it be your will, my Jesus, give me peace within. I need people around me. I need to be useful and busy. Give me the grace and the ability to live a productive life. Give me the strength to live out my life in surrender to your will. Amen

In time, things worsened. Mom craved people around her, but was also fearful of what she might say and do, afraid of the repercussions if others knew where her mind was. Her friends loved her, cared for her, and were concerned for her. I wonder if she had been open with them and shared her fears, anxieties, and worries, would that have relieved some of the pressure she put on herself? Her friends knew without having to be told because it was so obvious.

Her behaviors at the dinner table were interesting. She would pick things out of her plate. Usually we just let her be, but one day I just had to ask her what she was picking out of her plate. As calmly as possible, she replied as she continued eating, "I am taking out all of the bugs." She also had strange behaviors with her utensils. More than once she wrapped the utensils in the cloth napkin gently and gently lift it over to her shoulder, tapping the back of the napkin and rocking as if she were holding a baby. Even after Mom went into a facility, she would wrap her utensils. She usually would take them back to her room with her or put in her pocket. I don't know what she could have been thinking. Perhaps she was trying to clean up and didn't know where to put them?

Mom was part of a book club with ladies from her church. They would pick her up and bring her to the book study. They let her talk even though she didn't always make sense. They saw and loved the Beverly she was inside, the woman that was so filled with kindness and compassion towards others. They overlooked her deficiencies.

There was a couple that went out to eat with Mom and Dad every Monday, and sometimes on the weekends. It didn't matter that her hair wasn't washed, that she hadn't bathed in weeks, that her clothes were inside out and backwards. They simply showed unconditional love to her. Her friends never did abandon her, but they were the hands and feet of Christ to Mom in her time of need. No, she was never abandoned. She may not have recognized it, but Christ was always with her in her friendships. Christ sheltered his daughter daily, despite her struggles.

Mark 12:27
> He is not the God of the dead. He is the God of the living.

My Jesus, thank you for the gift of recognizing you in the

Something's Wrong; People Notice

everydayness of my life. Continue to allow the Spirit of your love to grace me with desire to know you and to act on that love and inspiration. It is such an enriching gift of your presence. Help me Lord to have focus and if it be your will, improve my memory. Amen

Luke 22:42
>Not my will, but your will be done

My Jesus, help me to be focused on your will for me. Give me the grace to recognize you in all things, to give my heart to follow your way. Lord, I need help with all of this. Give me your grace and love to follow you in all things. If it be possible, clear my head of all bad. Most of all Lord do not let my inability to reason hurt anyone.

Devotion

How do I recognize Christ in the everydayness of my life? I rush around going about my day. I see a multitude of people during the day, at work, in the store, on the road. I see them, but do I really look at them? Do I look beyond the ordinariness and risk reaching out of myself and my world to focus into others around me, focus on what they may be struggling with, or celebrate their joys with them?

My God is a God of the living. (Matthew 22:32) Am I really living if I am consumed only with my needs, my concerns, and my desires? I am called to fellowship with others and share the message of love Christ offers. When I take a step back from myself I can get a fresh look at a situation and recognize God's grace in the circumstance. I am so blinded by obstacles to grace, but another can see more clearly and guide me out of the mire I am bogged down in. I can do that for others. I am reassured God will give me the grace and love that I need to follow Him, every day.

Below is a letter Mom wrote to one of her oldest, dearest friends. The date is unknown. I am unsure if this was ever sent to her friend. Mom rarely spoke of her disease aloud, not even to her beloved husband, Paul. Her friend has remained her friend and still visits mom from time to time.

Friend,

I have always had a great respect for you. Last weekend was a very pleasant experience with your family here with us. I regret Paul was unable to be here. I know that your feelings were hurt by something I said. It was something that came out without any thought. You must also know that I have Alzheimer's. I understand that words sometimes come out that have not been thoughts. I regret that what came out of my mouth was an unkind one. I was as shocked as you were. It's the first time that this has happened. I'm sure it was painful for you to hear. I too was shocked. I am struggling with fear. I question, "Is this what I'm to battle in my future?" Please accept my apology. It was not my words. It was those of an evil me. Please pray for me. I know that you have always have been very close to our Lord. Again, please forgive me.

Devotion

Mom knew her actions where unacceptable but somehow

wasn't able to stop them. She calls it "an evil me." That is what sin is. We are human, imperfect sinners. Mom followed scripture in her response. She repented, regretted her actions, and asked for forgiveness. She knows this is the road back to Christ, because Jesus forgives all of our sin, no matter how ugly it may be. This is the way she can be whole again, to stay on track. With sin, we miss the mark, we go off road. We've missed where Christ wants us to be, the way Christ wants us to act. She questions if this is what her future holds? If I am open to listening to God, can I hear him warning me when I might be following the wrong path? In some instances, I am given the opportunity to heed the warning, make changes or change roads, before it messes up my life. In other cases, the warning may be there to help me cope with struggles I do not see that I will face in the future.

Mom starts experiencing behavior that is out of character for her:

12/9/2008

My Jesus, please help me to be calmer in stressful situations. My reaction yesterday was so out of character for me. Lord, I felt compelled to speak out. I felt disrespected, taken advantage of. We came with friends not to be manipulated, but enjoy the activity and each other. My peace has been shattered. Amen.

12/10/2008

My Jesus, I long to be healthy of mind, to have some memory and to be able to think rationally. If it be your will, my Jesus, take away the cloud, this mist in my head that keeps me from functioning properly. If this is your will, Lord, give me the grace to handle it. I long to be a good person. Give me the grace and fortitude to follow you my Jesus. I long to be a nice person and a peaceful person interiorly and exteriorly. Amen.

Devotion

How do I gain this confidence that God can piece back together a shattered life? It sounds so easy to live above your circumstances, have faith, and God is with you. It is so difficult to live out. Communication seems to be the key. Continuous, uninterrupted communication with Christ will do it. The Bible calls it "praying without ceasing" (1 Thessalonians 5:16-18).

Prayer is just talking to God. He knows everything anyway, so why not talk to Him about every aspect of your day, including your feelings. The ultimate goal is to stay in touch with Christ throughout the day, so He can guide your every step. Why do we instead act as if the goal is to be in control or to try to fix the situation?

Mom and Dad went to Mass or Bible Study 5-6 days a week, usually early mornings. The members in one of the groups would take turns preparing breakfast and leading the study. In the beginning, Mom was excited and creative in making breakfast dishes. Her breakfast casseroles were a favorite. As time went on, she could no longer put the ingredients together to make the casserole. She and Dad choose to purchase store-bought items

Something's Wrong; People Notice

such as frozen biscuit sandwiches. With the frozen items, all they needed to do was to heat them up in the microwave. Preparing food was one of the first activities Mom had trouble managing. It was easy to cover up her inadequacies by using frozen foods and fast food options.

This morning church group also took turns leading the devotion. Mom always thrived on preparing and finding the right scripture and apply meaningful understandings and applications for our lives from it. Again, there came a time when this was a struggle for her. She so much desired to keep sharing the message of Christ, but couldn't seem to get her thoughts together to have a cohesive message.

Instead of telling her no, Dad would find a daily devotional and give it to Mom as an inspiration knowing she could no longer prepare a devotion. She didn't even remember when it was her turn to prepare the devotion. The planning and preparation of things were no more. She just lived moment by moment. I had the opportunity to go with her and Dad one morning when Mom had to lead a devotion. Dad handed her a devotional book with the page bookmarked. She read over it at home right before we left as Dad instructed. When time came for her to lead, she read the devotion, but it was evident her reading skills had deteriorated. She struggled sounding out the words. Everyone at the table sat quietly and respectfully, not pointing out her mistakes. Specifically, there was a statement about how unique God created each of us. When she came upon the word "unique" she tried several times, without luck, until she asked for help. She commented, "Huh, I've never seen the word unique spelt before, interesting." She then continued reading the short devotion. She had nothing to contribute to the discussion after the reading.

Mom's struggles with being loved and wanting friendships seem to be getting stronger. She has begun to experience others avoiding her and becoming angry with things she has unintentionally said, yet she doesn't know how to mend the relationships and build on them.

1/2009

My Jesus, I am grateful for this time for myself, but, Lord, it seems like I need more to do to be productive. Please show me the path that you are calling me to. Volunteering for something would be nice, but could I do it? Heal me of my temper, my anxiety that overtakes me and drives me into unrest. Help me Jesus, to see you in all people. Teach me the way of loving detachment. I know what I would like to be, but I do not know how to achieve it. Please guide me. I long for good friends. That too, Lord, alludes me. I do have friends, but perhaps I do not know how to be a friend. Teach me empathy and compassion and when to act out of that. Give me purpose. I do have some disability, but I also have some capabilities. Show me how to be productive as long as possible.

1/2009

My Jesus, I need your grace your guidance, your intervention into that negative area of my brain. I long to be free of my negativity, my skeptic bias. Help me Jesus. I want to be a kind, considerate and loving person. Amen.

Medication was also an issue for Mom. Mom always lived a relatively healthy life and did not like to take medication unless it was absolutely necessary. Part of this stemmed from watching her own mother medicate daily for small aches and pains. She saw first-hand the consequences it can bring. Vitamins, on the other hand, seemed to be acceptable. Taking her medications

Something's Wrong; People Notice

became a battle for Dad. She would ask relentlessly what each pill was for. She would pick and choose which ones she wanted to take. There were many days, she refused to take her medicine or she thought she had already taken it. Often, she simply pushed them away saying she would take them later, but later usually didn't come. Dad would persist. Mom began calling him the "pill police." The inconsistency of taking her medication may have accounted for some of her behaviors.

2009

My Jesus, I want to be the person you want me to be. Please help me. Whatever it is that causes me to be mean, uncooperative, not understanding. Cleanse me of that meanness. I certainly did not intend to hurt or be mean to others, cause them pain or whatever. My Jesus, give me direction. Tell me what it is that you want me to do to bring reconciliation. I need a friendship base. I need friends as well as Paul's companionship. I put my life in our hands my Jesus. Tell me what to do. Amen.

2009

My Jesus, I long for inner peace, to trust completely in your will for me. I am so self-centered so much of the time. Help me to be more empathetic. I want to be more open and generous, but I'm not sure how to do that. I want friends, yet, I'm not sure how to do that either. Your Spirit Lord, infuse within me. Help me to see the goodness and the need in others. Give me the grace to know where it is you want me to be, what to do, and the movement of your Spirit guiding me in your direction and to speak your words for me. Lord, take away this fear of memory loss and negative behavior. Give me the spirit of loving. Amen.

An Introspective Journey

2/2009
Hebrews 1:12

> You will roll them up like a robe; like a garment they will be changed. But you remain the same, and your years will never end.

My Jesus, keep me focused on you. I have such confusion in my head from time to time. Please, Lord, heal me. If it is not your will for me to be stable in mind, give me the grace and spirit of being happy and kind to others. There is such a frustration in not being able to remember things along with fear of being misunderstood, discarded, avoided, laughed at, and abandoned. Thank you for your presence thus far. I should say the awareness of your presence. Show me how to be kind and loving. Give me the grace to be kind and loving.

3/17/2008
Daniel 3:42 (NABRE)

> But deal with us in your kindness and great mercy.

It is your kindness and love that gives me hope. As much as I want to be loving and kind, the more opportunity I find to practice love, forgiveness, and patience. I fail so miserably. This awful pessimism within me seems to be a block of cement around me, pulling me down. This brain thing is making me an unkind, mean person. I want to be kind and loving. I want to be accepted and respected as a human being. I long for self- worth, to really know I am accepted and cared for. And, Lord, whatever I have done to turn away my friends, I am truly sorry. I would like to know, even if it doesn't change things. And if it is my imagination help me to recognize that. If not, help me to accept and or correct whatever it is. Give me the grace Lord, to find my place in the community and in the church and with you. My Jesus, help me to find peace. Help me to find a place of indifference, knowing you are here with me. Amen.

3/23/2009

My Jesus,
Help me to find a true friend base. I know that my alienation from my friends is of my own making. Yet, Lord, my mental capacity was part of that rift. It seems to me that I have been sentenced without a trial. I am not sure that I understand what I perceive as a childish response. I would like to be able to be friends and do things with them, but part of me wants to distance myself from them. They have had some exposure to the memory losses and aging debilitations in their parents. Surely there is an awareness of memory loss and confusion as we age. Help me Jesus to handle and forgive for they know not what they do.

Help me Jesus in my acceptance of life and the pitfalls of aging. Walk with me my Jesus so that I will always do your will. Give me the grace to trust and walk in peace. Give me the gift of forgiveness and trust in your way for me. I thank you for opportunity to reflect on what I value and on what my value is. Rejection is one way to reevaluate what is important in my life. This I ask, my Jesus, that whatever becomes of these faltering relationships, let it be amicable.

I am saddened by this disconnect, but what is done is done. I have asked for forgiveness for my part in this; and I do realize that my forgetfulness is also a reminder to all that "this could be them" in fact may one day be them. I am sorry that compassion for the disability is not a part of their understanding. Perhaps it is the reality that "this could be me" that promotes anger and rejection. Help me Jesus to live with the awareness of a disability to forgive myself and others in their unawareness of disability. I have so much to be thankful for. Help me to focus on that. Thank you my Lord. Please do not abandon me. I trust. Amen. Beverly

3/26/2009

My Jesus, the message I hear today is awareness of your presence in all things. Trust in that presence. Live according to that presence. My Jesus, if it be your will, help me to find peace and to forgive myself for the crazy that comes out of me. Help me, Lord, to forgive those "friends" that turn their back on me, have not compassion for my disabilities. Help me, my Jesus, to be kind and loving. Help me to accept whatever it is my journey will bring me to. Be my companion, my Jesus. Guide me, counsel me, love me. Thank you for the opportunities to be with friends. Amen.

3/31/2009
Psalm 102:1-2

> Hear my prayer, Lord; let my cry for help come to you.
> Do not hide your face from me when I am in distress.
> Turn your ear to me;
> When I call, answer me quickly.

My Jesus these last few days my mind is filled with re-runs of things I have said and done that were childish and out of character; embarrassing myself and being out of control. The fear of losing my mind is a paramount. The things I say and do are not consistent with who I am normally. I have lost my friends and embarrassed myself to accommodate my behavior, my state

Something's Wrong; People Notice

of mind. My Jesus, help me to be kind. My behavior, even though I cannot help it, has cost me the companionship of friends. I ask forgiveness even though; I do not do it intentionally. My behavior has hurt others. I am sorry for that. It is not intentional, nor has it been done in malice. I thank you for Paul and his patience. Help him to cope with my craziness. If it be your will, my Jesus bring some stability to my life. Bless me with peace, acceptance of your will for me. Amen.

Dad is devoted to his wife and does everything he can to make things right, normal. He saw her behaviors, but he was met with much anger and fighting back because she believed she was right. She does not understand why he would "treat" her the way he does. Dad had to keep a close watch on Mom and couldn't leave her alone.

This posed a problem when they traveled. They would stop for lunch or coffee. Dad sat her at a table with her food. He'd instruct her not to move, but to stay there, explaining he was going to the bathroom and would be right back.

She was always "good" as Dad describes it. She listened and was obedient. He would give her instructions, then go to the restroom. When he returned he would direct her to go. He would wait at the door until she came out. Their life began to function in that way—Dad always watching out for her and giving her guidance. Many times prior to this she would exit the restroom before him. She was lost and didn't know what to do. Dad shared a story about an event that happened once at a stop. She left the restroom before he did. She searched for him and didn't see him and began to panic. When Dad came out she was running around frantically calling out his name. In her mind, she was alone, abandoned, lost.

Below are a few letters she wrote to him. The dates of the

letters are unknown. Eventually, Dad gives up on trying to help her understand her words and actions aren't speaking truth, due to the severity of consequences he endured. She did not only put her words on paper, but was very vocal in expressing her feelings to him.

> Paul,
> I do not know when I changed from being your wife and became your child. As an adult, I have the right to go to bed when I choose to among other things. Throughout our married life I have had the ability to live my life as I chose. For some reason here lately, you have chosen to expect from me your total direction for me. As far as I can recall the choices I have made have been adult and correct choices. I am very hurt that you feel like I have become your child and you should tell me what & how to do things. I don't always agree with the way you do things, but I respect that it's your way and its OK for you. It may not be the way I would do something, but you have the right to do things your way.
>
> But to expect me to do things as you perceive it to be the "only" right way (your way) is asking me to be someone else. I have spent many long days and nights with you working. It was I who saw to the children among other things. It was how we worked things out to fit our needs. What I did and said was accepted and trusted. Here lately I'm afraid to say what I think or believe because if it does not meet your expectations then I am criticized. I am who I am, nothing less. I spent many years with long days and nights on my own and with the children while you worked. I don't think I did a bad job with them.
>
> What is it about me that has become so unacceptable? I am not the woman you have made up in your mind I am supposed to be. I am Beverly with all my faults and you are Paul, my husband, with all your faults. All I can say to you is I am who I

am. I mean no harm for others. I don't always agree or embrace others' ideas and ways of doing things and by the same way that is how God made each person individual gifts and handicaps. I have never disgraced you. I treated you with respected and love. I don't have to agree with you to love you. I have always treated you with respect and love even when I disagree with what you say or do. I just thought that I had that same respect from you. I guess I am wrong. I am not to supposed to have ideas that are opposite from yours, but I do. I have that right. If what I say is so offensive to you, maybe we can communicate in other ways. I have just about decided that if we do not speak our personal ideas, then things can be closed. All I ever expected was to love and accept me as I am. Not as you would make me. Perhaps you have married the wrong person. I am who I am, warts and all. You just want to believe that you do not have any. We all have warts. We are called to love even the warts.

Beverly

Paul,
I am very hurt to think that after all these years together you have decided that who I am is not good enough for you. I am not you. I do not think like you. I don't always agree with what you say and do, but I still respect you for your beliefs and your appraisal of others and situations. I have been under the understanding that what I say or comment on in my own home to someone who professes to love me would be respected for what it is and just a comment. I see that I am wrong. I did not know that I had to get your approval of my feelings and observations of people and situations. You may not agree with my assessment, but it certainly is what I am reading into our comments.

For over 40 years I believed that you cared about time for who I am. Now, I find out that I was wrong. You expect me to be *whatever it is you expect of me, not who I am. If I cannot speak out to you how I am feeling about something who then am I to speak to?? This is my home. I expect to say what I am thinking out loud at times you have been very direct, not only this comment, but others over this past year especially, letting me know that I am not good enough for you.*

I am very hurt, that I am not loved by you as I have always thought you loved me. You are always making nice comments about others, not much praise for me. Yes, I am jealous. I want to be highly regarded by you. I am sorry that I am not your model person. I am pretty sure that I never was. I did hope that I was special, very special to you. I even thought I was, but, lately it is very obvious that is not so. I cannot be what you want. I can only be me. I do not want to live alone, but living alone would be better than living with someone who dislikes so much of what I do and say. I long to be your special one, I even find myself jealous of those people who you are always nice to and happy to be with.

It is obvious that you are not happy to be with me. I'm very sad about that, but I am who I am. You must decide if I am who you want.

Devotion

The agony Dad must have experienced living through this must have been incredible. What love he must have for his precious bride to put up with these blasts of anger that she hurled at him. That makes me think of another that suffered much agony being accused of things he did not do, and things he did not say. They didn't only hurl insults at him, but physically beat him, whipped him, and hung him up to die. He could have walked away, but he didn't. He didn't because of his love for you and me. Do I have the strength to love this way, unconditionally?

4/1/2009
Exodus 20:5

> You shall not bow down to them or worship them; for I, the Lord your God, am a jealous God, punishing the children for the sin of the parents to the third and fourth generation of those who hate me.

My Jesus, today's reading about is about the refusal to worship a false god speaks to me in my quest to deal with the rejection of my so-called friends. My loyalty is to rely on my God to trust that in some way I am being cared for even in the fire. The fire of rejection, lack of empathy one would expect of a friend. Knowing I have done this alienation to myself, but not intentionally. I told the truth, apologized for my error, yet, I am not forgiven. Instead I have been ostracized. They have turned their back on me. The years of friendship have been disregarded, the fact that this has never happened before.

That illness may have triggered all this. But, yes, I did neglect my responsibility, but to intentionally ignore me leaves me room for repentance or forgiveness. So, I guess, my Jesus, that if healing is to take place and forgiveness, you Lord, will have to intercede. Heal me, also help me to forgive myself and to move on. If it be in your will, Jesus, send people in my life that can support and encourage me to trust in others. Other misery, I'm looking at some very lonely times. Amen.

An Introspective Journey

4/5/2009
Isaiah 50:6

> I offered my back to those who beat me, my cheeks to those who pulled out my beard; I did not hide my face from mocking and spitting.

My Jesus, these last few months I have felt persecuted because of my failure with the ladies' retreat. Also, because of my memory deficits. My friends have turned their backs on me. I have been rejected as a person. I have no recourse. Because of me Paul too is being rejected because we are no longer "good" enough for these so-called friends. Help me Jesus see your hand, your compassion, and love. This deficit of memory is not of my making. Give me the grace of presence of mind to always react with kindness and love toward my persecutors. You, Lord, know how it feels to be rejected by those who claim to be our friends. Help me, my Jesus, to cope with whatever you send to me in my life. Heal me, Lord in whatever way I need healing. Give me a loving and forgiving heart and open arms to embrace you in all your faces. Amen.

Mom was so gifted and talented, but she was getting to the point that she wouldn't express herself because she feared rejection. She feared what people would think and tried to be perfect. Since no one is perfect, we will fall short. Our perception of ourselves can and often does get in the way of being as productive as we can be. Mom fell into that trap often and prayed to get out of her "pity pot."

I am the same way in wanting to be accepted and loved by others. I second guess myself in just about everything I say and do. Often I feel inferior to those around me, and my mind tells me that everyone knows how inadequate and worthless I am.

Something's Wrong; People Notice

The Bible tells me differently.

> "For you are my treasured possession."
> Exodus 19:5
>
> "I desire to establish you with all my heart and all my soul."
> Jeremiah 32:41
>
> "And I want to show you great and marvelous things."
> Jeremiah 33:3
>
> "If you seek me with all your heart, you will find me."
> Deuteronomy 4:29
>
> "For I am your greatest encourager."
> 2 Thessalonians 2:16-17
>
> "I gave up everything I loved that I might gain your love."
> Romans 8:31-32

Daily I must remind myself of these promises so that I don't fall into the trap of losing self-confidence. Many people in the Bible also felt less than qualified in doing God's work such as Moses, Jeremiah, David, and Jesus' disciples.

My flaws remind me that none of us were mass produced, but were fearfully and wonderfully made in the image of our creator. He made me different from others and that is what makes me special, not inferior. Mom took comfort in knowing that even Jesus felt rejection from his friends. I, too, must learn from Jesus.

Romans 8:31
> He came to demonstrate that I am for you, not against you.

4/6/2009

"Gratitude shouldn't be an occasional incident but a continuous attitude."

-Anthony Nyuiemedy-Adiase

Luke 17:15

One of them, when he saw he was healed, came back, praising God in a loud voice.

"I know not why God's wondrous grace to me. He hath made known; nor why, unworthy Christ in love Redeemed me for His own."

From the hymn: I Know I Have Believed"

My Jesus, so often I get into my pity pot, poor me! I long to be accepted, to be liked, well thought of. I want to do the right thing. However, it seems I do not know the right thing. As time goes on, I have less and less friends. My behavior becomes offensive to others, even when it is not meant to be. My Jesus, please help me to be more thoughtful of others, to be content with what is, to live in the moment. Help me to die to self for the sake of the others. Help me to recognize the right response to a situation, to see the good in all things first to love others because you love all. Help me to see the good first and to stop there, to be grateful for what is. My Jesus, forgive me for those times I am not kind and loving. Give me the grace to recognize my misbehavior. I ask you, Lord, for the grace to be forgiven and accepted by my "used to be" friends. I do not know what it is I can do more to repair my friendship with my friends. Forgive me for whatever I have done that alienated them. Heal me Jesus, if at all possible. I want to have good friends. I don't know how to change me. My Jesus, my life is in your hands. Let your Spirit of love that we celebrate or commemorate this week permeate my heart and soul. Change me

Something's Wrong; People Notice

Lord from self-serving to serving others; however, that is to be lived out. Give me the grace of a changed heart.

Mom had times she could feel that something wasn't right. She would know that she had said or done something to offend but didn't recall what that might have been. More than once, she would come and ask if she had said or done anything to offend me because she felt something was off. She would apologize for whatever she had said or done. Sometimes she had said or done something, but other times, there was nothing. She tried so hard to fix what she thought might be wrong. Perhaps she was so consumed in worry of offending others, she immediately thought she had. She was sharp in picking up moods, feelings, and reading the atmosphere around her. Somehow she knew something wasn't right, she knew there were missing pieces, but couldn't put it all together. Knowing her mind played tricks on her, she assumed she was in the wrong. This must have done a number on her self-esteem and confidence.

Devotion

Like so many of us, Mom's struggle was from within. She desperately wanted to be kind and compassionate but knew there were times she did not act this way. We all have times when waves of emotions take over our actions. We all strive to manage our emotions positively because of how it effects the way we relate with others.

An Introspective Journey

Romans 7:15

> I do not understand what I do. For what I want to do I do not do, but what I hate I do.

She knew the way to reconciliation when something didn't feel right. Forgiveness melts away walls and obstacles that trap us. Reconciliation reunites people back together. It is about restoring relationships.

Where is my focus? Do I think more about myself and my point of view than about others? How often do I miss opportunities to reconcile relationships because of my stubborn pride holding on to how I was wronged?

Romans 12:18-21 clearly describes what I should do:

> [18] If it is possible, as far as it depends on you, live at peace with everyone.
>
> [19] Do not take revenge, my dear friends, but leave room for God's wrath, for it is written: "It is mine to avenge; I will repay," says the Lord.
>
> [20] On the contrary: "If your enemy is hungry, feed him; if he is thirsty, give him something to drink. In doing this, you will heap burning coals on his head."
>
> [21] Do not be overcome by evil, but overcome evil with good.

She researched all she could about Alzheimer's Disease but did not discuss it with others. She acted on "home remedies" that were suggested to improve memory. Knowing that keeping the brain active was recommended, she played "brain games."

One game she played for a long time was Spider Solitaire. She challenged herself to work up to three suites in solving the game. She had a laptop and played it almost daily when she had the chance.

When she heard coconut oil would slow the progression, she took that. She tried other over the counter remedies and vitamins that may help her. Invariably, she did anything that sounded reasonable in an effort to slow this disease. She always talked about wanting to participate in a study about Alzheimer's Disease since it was prevalent on both her maternal and paternal sides. She never could bring herself to do this. Perhaps after the caregiving for her parents was over, she was too afraid given her memory issues to seek a definite answer. Perhaps it was too much for her to bear.

Out of respect and my desire to seek a cure for those struggling with this disease, I have, like other siblings in my family, participated in studies to help with this. I was asked why I wanted to put myself through the physical tests and procedures involved. I could only say that I could not help my mom overcome this disease, but didn't want anyone else to have to live with it either. If there was anything I could do to help find a way to avoid this, I was all in.

Look online, ask at the doctor's office. There are so many studies and with help from people like us, we are getting closer to figuring out how to rid this world of this horrendous disease that is growing and slowly taking the lives of our loved ones.

Devotion

Aren't we all searching for answers? Does finding the "answer" hold the key to finding happiness and contentment? There's nothing wrong with searching for ways to make things better, but we can't let that overwhelm and overtake our lives. There are times I am so consumed in a project or situation, that life doesn't happen. I become filled with anxiety and worry about the future I forget to live in the now. I don't want to miss out on the now. God has this, He has me and my future. Regardless what happens, I am not alone.

I am assured that Christ will care for me. I count on Him and hold on to Him at the center of my being to bring me through the hard times I must face. But Christ is also counting on me to share my life with others. He is counting on you too. Each of us has a purpose that we must fulfill. No longer can we wallow in self-pity, but must look for how to share the love of Christ every day. We need each other as the body of Christ for encouragement and support. Today, I will look around and find someone that I can encourage and support.

9/2009
Luke 1:77

> To give his people the knowledge of salvation through the forgiveness of their sins, because of the tender mercy of our God, by which the rising sun will come to us from heaven to shine on those living in darkness and in the shadow of death, to guide our feet into the path of peace

My Jesus, I so often find myself in darkness. I am overwhelmed with concern to what our future holds. I desire to be useful to others and especially to Paul. I long for good friends with to care about me. I long for laughter and fun times. Help me to be grateful for all.

Something's Wrong; People Notice

10/2009

I long for clarity and presence to the moment. To make sense in my conversations. I long to be accepted just as a human being, just as I am. Jesus, I beg you to bring clarity into my mind. Give me the grace to forgive myself and others who seem to get so bent out of shape by me. Thank you, my Jesus, for your presence in my life and thank you for Paul. Help me to always recognize the gift that he is to me. Give me the direction I need in my life to continue the journey to you. You know all the pain I feel inside of me. You know the peace I long for. My Jesus, grant me that inner peace. Amen.

11/8/2009

My Jesus, this weekend has been very telling for me. One thing I realized, I do not have many true friends. But it gives me a new freedom knowing this. I know to lower my expectations of them. The best for me is that I can stand in indifference with it all. There may come a time when I will be unable to do much. But, with your help can have a happy life. I continually come back to "indifference." Ignatius standing in the middle and trusting God's guidance. For one thing falling into step with you Lord is the best thing I can do. Continue to guide me Lord. Help me to accept whatever you have in store for me. If possible, Lord, give me friends that accept me as I am. Like my friend who is so very special. "Father, as you said on the cross, your will be done." One more request, Lord. Remind me to journal. It really is helpful. Thank you brother Jesus for being you. Love, Beverly

Alzheimer's advocate Meryl Comer says the following: "Nothing prepares you for this disease. No one is prepared for the isolation. Friends disappear because the person they knew is no longer there. The caregiver gets trapped with the patient. It is very lonely and isolating."

Despite all the journal entries about rejection from her friends, it was not evident by others around her. She continued going to church daily for Mass or Bible Study. She went places with other ladies during this time. She felt that disconnect internally but had not been rejected outwardly by her friends although they could see what was happening to her. They also did not know the truth of the conflicts going on inside her and how hard she fought to prevent her memory and her life functioning. Her friendships did decrease, maybe it was from the wall Mom put up in an attempt to keep others from knowing her secret or perhaps it was the embarrassing behaviors Mom displayed in public or the way she did not take care of herself without bathing or changing her clothes.

At church, she taught a class on Spiritual Direction. Since she had taught it for several years, she knew the information well. As the years passed the material became harder and harder to retrieve and present. It was painful to watch as she prepared. She read the chapters over and over, taking notes on what to emphasize. She practiced speaking in an empty room, wanting so much to get it right.

I recall her returning from a class one evening, disappointed because things did not go well. I didn't completely understand. She knew the material and had presented it many times before and she had practiced over and over to get it right. At the time I was baffled as to why she needed to practice so many times. I thought perhaps it wasn't as bad as she described. She had to give up this ministry that meant so much to her.

Mom studied the life of St. Ignatius of Loyola. He articulated beneficial guidelines for the discernment of spirits. She examines

Something's Wrong; People Notice

herself and how she trusts God's guidance. Her spiritual maturity was nourished by continually learning, attending workshops, seminars and continuing education. It is so clear that her goal was to grow closer to Jesus and to live her life doing what she could to bring others closer to Him.

2/2/2010

Today the weather is wet and chilly. I am excited to see new things and places. Please, Lord, give us dry and warm weather. Help me Jesus to open to you as we go through these next 10 days. I so long to be a part of a group who like and respect me as who I am. Help me to be less sensitive to being or feeling rejected by others. Help me to remember. I try to the best of my ability, to be kind and respectful to others. All I want is to have good friends who care about me and respect me as I am. Give me the grace to be kind and respectful and to have a good relationship with people, especially by those that I respect and care about.

My Jesus, be my guide and my mentor. I long for good close friends. Help me to discard all that is not life giving.

2/2010

My Jesus, I have spent a lot of time and energy to fit in and to be liked by others. It has occurred to me that you are the one I want to please. Help me, Jesus, to be respectful to others and to be reminded that you are the one I want to be accepted by. Help me Lord to be kind and respectful to others and to always respect all, because we are all your children. Help me Lord to look for your guidance and your love for me. I cannot change how others see me. Teach me to always be respectful to all even when I am hurt and rejected. Be my guide and my protector. Amen

An Introspective Journey

The disease might hide the person underneath, but there's still a person in there who needs your love and attention – Jamie Calandriello

Mom's journal writing end here. She could no longer put thoughts together and difficulty putting letters together to make a word. Even these last few journal entries were difficult to read. Her handwriting changed, her spelling off. For example, she would do things like use a "g" instead of a "q." Her letters were poorly formed. One entry she referred to Mother Teresa. She spelt "Mother Teresa" as "Muther Theresa."

She had several notebooks around and wrote in whichever was closest to her when she wanted to write. I found notebooks in her prayer room, in her side table by her bed and on the end table in the living room. She randomly put things in the notebook. Once I found in the back of a notebook, upside down, my name, "Paula." Beside it, she wrote, "my daughter's name." I wonder, was she trying to remember?

It wasn't long before more people began noticing something just wasn't right. By this time, she let go of her responsibilities. Volunteering at church became more difficult. There came a time the church asked her to stop reading scripture during the service. She wrote a letter to the priest expressing her disappointment and hurt clearly not understanding why they would stop her from her service to the Lord. She did not share this with Dad. She told him she had decided she did not want to do it any longer. The letter she wrote revealed she was covering up for her inadequacies and embarrassment.

Preparing food continued being a challenge. We knew when we visited, we would have refrigerator biscuits for breakfast, usually burnt. Sometimes, they picked up a can of cinnamon rolls to fix, which was a treat. Mom would put them on the pan and

Something's Wrong; People Notice

with help, get them into the oven to bake. When the biscuits and cinnamon rolls were done, I watched as she took the icing from the package and squeeze a dab on each biscuit and cinnamon roll, then threw the leftover icing away. She would not accept help and would become angry if she felt anyone questioned anything she was doing. Many many times, she stomped to the back of the house, slammed her bedroom door closed and talked with Dad because she felt she had been wronged in some way.

2011

Some time during this year, Mom went to the doctor expressing her struggle with coping. The doctor did add Namenda to the Aricept she was already taking. This was kept very quiet to the family. Nothing more than an acknowledgment of "having a little bit of dementia." She never talked about what she was experiencing, even with Dad. Dad's concern was increasing. Although Mom still had a cell phone, she never used it. Most days, it was left at home. Dad did not have text messaging on his phone, but with encouragement, he later added it. This was a blessing for us. For the first time he had a means to reach out for help without her knowledge. It was a big step for him when he canceled her phone line. She never even noticed.

2012

As the years went on, Mom needed more people around her all the time. There came a time when she refused to even go to a restaurant with just Dad. She would only go if someone else joined them.

The biggest problem is that Mom could no longer cook. She spent her life cooking for her family and thought she was able, but wasn't. This was a difficult struggle for Dad. He figured out how to go out to eat and take home leftovers for the next day. I can't imagine what his credit card bill looked like each month with dinner out almost nightly. Even ordering at a restaurant would be tricky. She either could no longer read, or didn't understand the options. At first, she would talk about options she could get, and order that way. Later she would point to something to the waiter. Often she was surprised and sometimes upset when her order came because she didn't believe she had order that item.

Quite often, Dad ordered a cup of gumbo before his meal. He would ask her if she wanted one. She usually said no, but would become angry with the waiter if Dad got a cup and she didn't. Eventually, Dad ordered for her what he ordered. This kept the peace.

There were times I would visit when she would allow me to cook. Most of the time, she tried to help. I had to watch her closely and do my best to make sure things were cooked correctly. Many times, I'd have to go behind her back and correct something she had done. I'd take the leftovers and freeze it for Mom and Dad to have later. The next time I visited, I noticed the frozen food was still there. I asked Dad why they had not eaten what was in the freezer. Dad said mom could not figure out how to heat it up and she wouldn't let him help her. So, they went out to eat.

Cleanliness was an issue. Family and friends had to be careful with the dishes we ate and drank from. Mom was always in motion, loading and unloading dishes. She could not tell when the dishes were clean. She often put dirty dishes back in the cabinets. Dad no longer had the energy to argue. The combinations of foods she fixed were odd. Foods that should have been heated weren't and foods that should have been cold were heated. It did not matter, Dad ate what she gave him on whatever dish she served it in.

The same is true about her clothes. She would wear the same clothes day after day. She confused which machine was the washer and which was the dryer. It would not be uncommon to find detergent in the dryer or for her to dry her dirty clothes and wear them again believing they were clean. She never seemed to notice stains on her shirt.

10/2013

This disease hits hard when there is extra stress on the patient. We were jolted into reality when Dad had knee replacement surgery in October 2013. Mom was at his side, although very confused at the hospital. The plan was for her to sleep there with him since Dad did not feel comfortable leaving her at home by herself.

We didn't realize the state she was in and with her independent nature, decided to drive home one evening while he was in the hospital. Since the nurses were aware of her confusion, they called a family member informing the family that she had left. It took Mom much longer than it should have to get home, but she made it. Once she got home, my sister was there. Mom couldn't even figure out how to find the right key and get it into the door to unlock it.

Once inside, she began calling friends looking for Paul. She eventually called is cell phone angrily, demanding he come home immediately. Her memory of the day had left her. The following day at the hospital, she spoke with me expressing her concern for her "father," who she believed was who was in the hospital. Her concern was that this man claimed to be her husband, Paul. She was determined to prove to "her father" that he was wrong. It was later discovered that with all the chaos, she had not taken her medication. Perhaps things would have been different had she taken her medicine. We are not sure. We will never really know.

Once dad was released, I was with them for some recovery time at their home. My observations were that she quickly became agitated often believing something was accurate when it wasn't. I found items in strange places, like a box in the freezer. She must be followed, which Dad had been doing, to find where she was placing things.

She didn't fully understand his condition or how to properly care for him such as how to change his bandage. Once I observed her carefully wrap his foot instead of his knee with an ice pack. Dad didn't have the heart to tell her she was doing anything wrong. She asked him to get up and do things such as make her some coffee, get the mail, or go to the store, clearly not realizing this was not possible with his knee surgery. It was during this week I emphasized to Dad the seriousness of not allowing her to drive. In his mind, she would be OK if he was there telling her where to go. Dad did not understand that she could forget how to drive, no matter how much we told him. He did allow her to drive him to his doctor appointments before he was released to drive again. I thank God for His protection at this time. When Dad was able to drive again, he no longer let her drive. This wasn't too big of an obstacle because dad usually did all the driving and she never asked.

One morning I overheard an argument between her and Dad. I wish this had been a one-time argument, but this was common and happened often. She accused him of having a child with another woman. She was certain that several people had told her so. He was unable to convince her this was not true. She kept saying it was his word against all the others. It was intense. She was so sure she was right. Dad offered her to call whomever

Something's Wrong; People Notice

she wanted to clear things up. She refused. I broke in the conversation, changing it and she quickly forgot the conversation. I wonder how many times did Dad have to suffer through these accusations?

There were times Dad would call out of the blue and ask me to call Mom. Other times he called for her. She would ask where my children were because she believed they were at her house, but couldn't find them. Sometimes, she thought my children were at my sister's house and wanted them to come back to her house. The same scenario happened with my brother and his family who lived in Florida.

Once, when staying at her house, she asked me who the lady was that was sleeping at her house. I told her it was me. She insisted there was someone else there. She did this often now, not recognizing family in her home or believing someone is there that is not. She no longer remembers having some of her grandchildren or that all of her children are married.

Many times after this when I visited, she would tell Dad she was uncomfortable with "this situation." When he asked her "what situation" she told him she was uncomfortable with this woman who was with them saying she was their daughter.

She also asked me who the young girl was that came to borrow her computer. No one had.

Mom was always active and desired to be on the go continuously. She and Dad often traveled with others. There was a trip they went on with her son's in-laws. During the trip, Dad had been dropped off somewhere, but Mom stayed in the car toward the next destination. It was during this time, Mom kept forgetting where Dad had gone. She repeatedly panicked thinking they had "forgotten Paul." They had to remind her multiple times that Dad was safe and explain the situation to her.

They would come to Tennessee to visit us when they could.

An Introspective Journey

I overheard her tell Dad one day when they were visiting me, "Paul, it's time for you to pay the lady." Dad was puzzled and asked, "What lady?" She answered, "The lady that let us stay here. We have to pay for our stay. It is time to go home." I was not her daughter at this time, but just a kind lady that let her stay in her home.

Stories like these became more frequent. Knowing how to react and respond is difficult. It is so strange and off. I can understand why so many family and friends become distant or angry with the person with Alzheimer's.

Chapter 8

Getting Help

2013

Mom was no longer able to care for herself. Grooming habits were minimal. She would go weeks without a bath and longer without washing her hair. Dad had no one guiding him on how to handle this situation. She would become angry when he would make a suggestion to bathe. There were times; she would turn on the water, then turn it off, not realizing she hadn't even gotten in the shower. Other times, she did get in the shower, but after getting wet, would get out without washing her body.

Dressing was also a struggle. Physically she could dress herself, but her clothes no longer matched. Sometimes she wore Dad's pants or shoes. Often her clothes were backwards, inside out and most of the time, dirty.

Getting her to the beauty salon was a challenge. No matter what tactics Dad tried, he could not get her to go. When family came to visit, we would have a "girls' outing" to the beauty shop. Mom would come to be with us, but insisted she did not need a haircut. When we got to the shop, we all had a turn, sometimes in the chair next to her and got our hair or nails done. This worked most of the time, but there were still times she refused. We were lucky if we got her hair cut every six months. It is challenging to get someone to do something they don't want to or see a reason to do something they don't think needs to be done.

Mom would not allow Dad to clean anything. She would stop him, saying she planned to get to it later. Later never came. The sheets on their bed were stained yellow and smelled, but nothing was touched. There even came a time when Dad got the sheets off the bed, but could not get them back on. I am not sure how long they slept in a bed without sheets or pillowcases. For the sake of peace, Dad let things be unless there was any potential harm to her.

The strain on Dad was mounting. Mom always wanted to go somewhere. Besides telling him where to turn and then fussing at him when he didn't, the rides in the car seemed to be calming for her. Years later, Dad confessed there were times when he thought it would be easy to veer into the oncoming traffic and have a head-on collision. He said they could die together and both be at peace. It was just a thought because he could never do anything to hurt her or anyone else. He carried the guilt of not being able to care for his wife properly. The burden of wanting to fix everything was high, but there was nothing he could do to make it right. Watching her was breaking his heart with seemly nowhere to turn to for help. He too must have done a lot praying and felt alone much of the time.

Dad struggled to get information to the doctor. What a challenge that was. He was trapped. He was the only one who really knew the truth of what was happening to his beloved. She watched every step and listened to every call. She is around him around the clock, 24 hours a day, even following him when he goes to the bathroom. He was a prisoner in this situation. When they visited the doctor and was asked how things were going, he could do nothing but tell the doctor everything was

Getting Help

OK. He longed for the doctor to look up and see him nodding his head "no," while he couldn't bring himself to say it aloud, at least not in front of her.

For quite some time, she was a master at social graces with the doctor and with those she had short conversations with. She sounded believable unless she talked longer. Finally, in December 2013, Dad gave me permission to communicate with the doctor on his behalf. I expressed how we saw Mom's mind working as if things that happened in the past are in the present. How she is anxious and in constant motion, not sitting still. I told him of her emotions being up and down all day long. How she gets angry over things that have not happened and confronting people for things she believes are true. The doctor heard how Dad gets the brunt of this. The doctor could not help us until he knew the truth of the situation. Even though Mom and Dad needed this help for a long time, it wasn't until things got beyond rough that Dad had the courage to seek help. They lived with this "secret" of denial of this disease that had infested into all parts of their lives. Even living in these conditions, Dad did not have the courage to share his struggles with the doctor himself. Slowly he shared bits of what was happening with me. I am no counselor and did not always know the best way to handle things. But someone had to handle it for him. It wasn't until I was able to intervene on his behalf that we could seek more appropriate medical care for Mom.

The doctor sent us to a neurologist who specialized with these types of behaviors. This doctor gave her the diagnosis of Alzheimer's Disease after a thorough examination that included a brain scan. All the hallmarks of the disease were there. Mom and Dad chose not to share this diagnosis openly with the family. Her medication was adjusted. Even with this doctor, Dad was unable to communicate the truth of what was happening every day. Dad felt comfortable enough sharing his daily trials with me. But I couldn't talk with him daily, privately, or depth of what was actually happening at home. Mom watched his every step and listened to every call. With her paranoia, if she wasn't with him in everything, she thought the worst.

As doctor appointments occurred, I encouraged Dad to share what he was experiencing in her behaviors at home. He would not. He couldn't bear to speak aloud what was happening. I am not sure if it was that he was too embarrassed to speak of the happenings or if he were too afraid to say them in front of Mom. Dad never took the opportunity to talk to the doctor in confidence privately without Mom with him. When the doctor asked how things were going, Mom responded "no problems, everything is fine." Dad would shake his head behind the doctor, who didn't always notice. He didn't speak up, and his struggles continued. Oh, how frustrating it was for us, their children, to have such high hopes that things could get better after the doctor appointment, but time and time again, they would come away with nothing new because they would not tell the truth of the situation. One of the first times he recognized how significant her disease was when the neurologist asked mom some simple questions and had her do some simple exercises. The day at the doctor's office when Mom could not draw a complete circle and put in numbers to create a clock will forever be in Dad's mind. She couldn't answer straightforward, simple questions. For so long she talked around specifics, Dad hadn't comprehend the depth of her illness.

Dad loves his wife and does want to be with her, but misses her companionship. It has disappeared.

2014 Continued

Mom is confused most of her days now but does everything

Getting Help

she can to disguise it. She is anxious and is continually on the move. Multiple times a day Mom would say something like this, "OK, I think it's time to go home." "I'm ready to go home." "Let's get our stuff and head home." She didn't realize it, but she was already home. She was longing for that place that is familiar, comfortable. That place she could completely relax. Think about never being able to go home, never being sure where each room was, what was around the corner. How would it feel to always be in an unfamiliar setting? Vacations and hotels are nice to visit, but there's nothing like coming home. Dad usually ignored her asking. He hoped it would either go away or that he would be able to distract her long enough for her to forget she was asking to go home. Some days, she would walk out the door and go sit in the car waiting for Dad until he "brought her home." His response was to get in the car and drive around until he drove back home. He can't seem to make it stop and doesn't know where to turn for help. He is surviving and can't do much more than that.

She is paranoid of people in her house and of her husband having an affair. She is angry and lets it out on Dad. It doesn't matter what he says; she will not believe or understand. It does not matter what proof he has to the contrary, she is not rational in her thinking. It becomes an endless cycle that he can't talk his way out of. He needs something to distract her from her thoughts. This is when text messaging becomes a lifesaver for Dad. He'd text for help from me. I'd call her and talk to her. She'd get distracted, thinking of other things and he'd have peace for a short time. The frequency of his texts increased. The effectiveness of distracting her did not work as well as it had previously.

As time moves forward, things worsen. When home, she frequently asks to go home. She makes comments about how she has a piece of furniture like the one "in this place she is visiting" at her own home. She refuses to believe she is at home. When asked where she lives, she would respond with various cities from the one she grew up in to the one where she currently lives. Regardless, she doesn't recognize the place is in as home. Although her answers are off-based, she is confident with her answers. There is no telling her she is incorrect. Correcting her is only makes her distrust you more because she can't comprehend why you would disagree when she is right.

Occasionally, she gets out a suitcase and packs for a variety of reasons. Sometimes it is to go home, sometimes to go on a trip, sometimes it is to leave her husband. She packs items that do not make sense. She includes her deceased mother's jewelry, paper, knickknacks, towels, shorts and perhaps a jacket.

There are days she would get angry or decide to go walking. Dad could not keep up because of arthritic knees but would try. They know a lot of folks in the neighborhood. Neighbors would see her walking and bring her home. Once we followed her at a distance with the car making sure she was safe. When possible, someone would walk with her. On one of those occasions when walking with her, she told me an elaborate story in great detail of a house she claimed Dad bought in the town she grew up in without her seeing it. If I had not known better, I might have believed her. She believed every word she said. She described the house and its location. She explained how and when Dad told her and showed her the house. She was quite upset with him for making such a decision without her although she did say she liked the house. Knowing how to respond to something so outrageous is difficult to say the least, especially when she believes to be true. The best I could do is to listen to her, recognize the feelings she was experiencing, and offer support without condemning what she believed was true.

In 2014, Dad was worn out. Dad needed support and the

Getting Help

doctor needed to know the entirety of her condition. Dad agreed to let me accompany them on a visit with the neurologist. This was a big step and one that Mom was not happy about. She did not see a need for me to be with her, but agreed with support from Dad. For the first time, I requested for Dad and me to see the doctor without Mom's presence. They worked it out for the nurse to stay with Mom in the room while Dad finally was able to be totally honest with the doctor about what was happening at home. The doctor understood and was supportive of Dad. When the doctor saw mom in his office, he asked her some basic questions. Most of which she could not answer correctly. She didn't know her birthday, the current day, or who the president was. It was evident something needed to be done. Again, medication was changed and adjusted.

I will never forget the mind boggling conversation in the car on the way home that morning. She held the "Summary of Today's Visit" in her hands. She was reading over it and becoming agitated. She waved the paper at me and exclaimed she now had proof from the doctor that there was nothing wrong with her, that she did not have Alzheimer's Disease and could prove it with this summary report. I just want to cry in awe because the first line in the report was the diagnosis: Alzheimer's Disease.

I felt relief that now things would change now that the doctors understood the scope of the situation. We had high hopes medication changes would make a difference. There was little change in her behaviors. What did change was Dad's willingness to seek help. He allowed me to be more involved in caregiving decisions. He still could not talk at length about things, but I took what he shared and researched ways to help them.

I made a point to share with Dad everything I did concerning Mom's care. Mom already had trust issues with others around her. Dad needed support and to know he was still making the decisions regarding Mom. He just didn't have the energy or ability to know where to go and what to do. When I made a suggestion, I did not act on it until he approved. Sometimes I had to remind him of specifics to get him to agree to certain help. One was to activate her long term care insurance and acquire home health to assist them in their home. Dad was not very keen on this idea at first, and I would not force it on him, but kept reminding him of the benefits.

Dad finally agreed to have home health come into their home to spend some time with Mom, so he could have some time to himself. He needed time to go to the store, pay bills, or simply sit quietly by himself. She was paranoid about everything he did and everyone he talked to. He could not go to the grocery store without her jumping on him when he returned because in her mind he took too long. Five minutes to her seemed like half the day. She would be furious with him for leaving her alone for so long.

More and more, he was afraid to leave her by herself, but she would often refuse to go with him. There were times he would have to leave her alone to go pick up food because she refused to go with him. During these times, he'd call me from his car. I'd call her at home and keep her on the phone until he came back, that is if she picked up the phone. I know there were times she tried "answering the phone" with the TV remote control. Many times he did convince her to go with him. Unfortunately, when he drove back into the driveway, she would refuse to get out of the car because she would not go into someone else's home. She did not recognize her own home.

Frantic phone calls came from Dad wondering what to do with her. She would just sit in the car as if he was dealing with business and would come back soon. I'd call the house to talk with her. When she heard I was on the phone for her, she would

Getting Help

come to answer and then forget she had been waiting in the car. All it took was a distraction from what she was doing, and she could return to some sort of normalcy.

As her behaviors intensified, Dad was unable to call me because he could not get away to talk. He would walk to the shed in the backyard to call from his cell when he needed to speak with me. He talked fast because it was not long before she'd followed him back there. He could not escape her to even get help. If he went to the back of the house, she followed him. She always wanted him to herself, not doing anything else. And that is what he did. He put down whatever he was doing and went back to the living room to sit on the couch with her.

Dad had bills that needed to be paid and errands to run. Some days, she would go with him to the store, but often refused to get out of the car, so dad left her in the car in the parking lot. What a blessing that she never got out and wandered around as so often Alzheimer's patients do.

Talking to her both on the phone and in person became difficult. She didn't know what to say. If asked what she had been doing, she would come up with a believable story of visiting with one of her friends or running errands. Mostly, these were just things to say, I suppose, hoping there was some truth in them. She honestly didn't know where she had gone or who she had been with.

Mom had a desire to be active. She is social and loved visiting with others. For the most part, she was good in the car. She was content knowing she was going somewhere.

When Mom and Dad weren't visiting with friends or family, driving around in the car, or at church, they sat in front of the television. There simply was nothing else Dad knew he could do with her. He was exhausted and needed to rest. The words from her journal about life in retirement saddens me.

An Introspective Journey

I am so afraid of retirement, yet, I want the freedom to do whatever whenever. Lord, give me some productive things to do. Give Paul some productive things also. Help each of us find our balance personal as a couple. Yesterday evening, we hardly spoke to each other, just watched TV. I'm saddened and longing for some excitement, some activity we could do together. I fear his retirement. What will be expected of me? Is all we will do be around the house?

I now wonder if she realized her fear of doing nothing was coming true or if her mind was elsewhere and never made that connection.

12/2014

Holidays were difficult for Mom. She loved having her family around and insisted on having everyone at her house. The noise and craziness of having so many people around exasperated her difficulties in coping with life. It was during these times that we saw more erratic behavior from her.

Her younger grandchildren did not have the opportunity to interact with her the way her older grandchildren did. They would be playing on the floor, and out of nowhere, she would fuss at them for disobeying her. She would go up to them and say, "How many times I have to tell you not to play here?" It was apparent she thought they were her children. They didn't know how to respond. One day she noticed the youngest grandchild playing in a tree in her backyard. He was probably around eight years old at the time. She was very worried about this strange child in her backyard and wondered if she should call the police to come get him. I distracted her from this thought, thinking all would be OK.

Getting Help

I was wrong. Her worry increased about this child. She later found him in the back of the house. She asked me to come with her as she confronted him. She called him over and asked him who his mom and dad were. With kindness and compassion, she explained to him she needed to call the police to come and get him, that everything would be OK. She was so kind and gentle in explaining things to him. He just looked at me in bewilderment and said nothing. I went to get my brother, his father. When we came back into the room she had her arm around him, comforting this lost child. When we told her this was her grandchild, I remember her being very hurt in finding out for the first time that her son had been married and had a child. She was sad, shaking her head and quietly saying "no one ever told me." Wanting at that time to do nothing but love her new found family members. She cried and held them close.

2/2015

Home health was not the answer for Mom. She needed so much more. Even the home health nurse said she could not believe Dad was able to hang on for as long as he had with her in this condition. I still remember her saying, "she's really far along in this disease." Mom became suspicious that every time this woman came over, Dad would leave. Mom begged him not to leave, so instead, he just went to the back of the house. Mom would come find him and ask him to come join her. She often complained that this lady wanted her to go places that she didn't want to go. She did go sometimes for a cup of coffee or a doughnut. Her behaviors were becoming more intense.

Mom didn't sleep well. Dad gave her a glass of wine every night at nine o'clock to help her fall asleep. She had nightmares and would scream in her sleep. Sometimes she wandered around the house. When Dad found her wandering, she was usually looking for someone that wasn't there. Once she was in a panic because she got up to check on "the baby." Imagine how concerned she was when she could not find "the baby." Dad wasn't sleeping well at night for fear that she would walk out of the house. He upgraded his home alarm system and put the beeps on the doors as loud as they could go. He thought he would hear the beep and wake up if she tried leaving. Thankfully, she never did try to leave in the middle of the night. Eventually, the home health nurse suggested we admit her into a behavior clinic to see if medication could be adjusted.

There is a moral task of caregiving, and that involves just being there, being with that person and being committed. Where there is nothing that can be done, we have to be able to say, "Look, I'm with you in this experience. Right through to the end of it." (Dr. Arthur Kleinman)

We were extremely nervous and anxious about placing her in the behavior clinic but did not know what else to do for her. It was very confusing to her, but she didn't argue. She never really understood where she was or why she was there. When asked she would say she was visiting with her cousins. Every evening we could visit her. During this visit, she argued on why she could not come home with us. Many times, she thought she was in a hospital taking care of one of her parents. Convincing her to stay was short lived. As soon as we would persuade her to stay, a few minutes later she was asking to leave again.

Dad has never been able to lie to Mom, no matter the circumstances. It was during this stay that he came to the realization that telling "white lies" to her could be for her own good. This is what happened. She asked where her mom was one evening during a visit. Dad told her the truth, that her mom had passed

Getting Help

and was no longer alive. It was evident in her facial expressions the hurt and sadness that rushed over her. In her mind, this was the first time she had heard this news. It was heartbreaking. Now when Mom asks about her parents, Dad changes the way he replies. Instead of saying they are dead, he says they are together, in the town where they lived. If Mom questioned him further, he would say the name of the funeral home, as if it was someone she would know. She has always accepted this explanation. Dad feels good he doesn't have to lie but would do so now if it means sparing her the pain and anguish she would feel if she knew the truth.

When visiting time was over, a nurse would have to walk her away from us because she would try to come along with us. Watching Dad's face as he would have to leave her and seeing the confusion on her face was almost unbearable. We had to keep telling ourselves, *We're doing this for her good.* The stay at the clinic was unsuccessful in tracking her erratic behaviors because she didn't display any unusual behaviors while in the clinic aside from confusion and roaming the halls. Instead, she was polite and on her best behavior. No medication changes were suggested. Even so, I don't believe this stay was totally unsuccessful. During her short stay, Dad had some time for some much needed rest. We were able to clean her house. The doctors and nurses had a family meeting before releasing Mom. For the first time, someone had evaluated mom's condition and made some surreal recommendations for her. They recommended moving her directly from the hospital setting to a facility.

This was more than Dad could take. He agreed to let us look at facilities together if, and when, the time came. He refused to "give up" on her. It was difficult to help him understand that helping her could mean putting her in a facility that could better meet her needs. Three of the four siblings were able to go with

Dad and look at places. We chose a place we felt she would be comfortable in and was put on a waiting list.

Family relations were strained as Mom's disease took over her. She believed my sister had it out for her and wanted to put her in an insane asylum. She confided in me her fear of the motives of my sister. Mom had a great distrust with anything my sister said and did. Mom thought the reason my sister had a desire to put her away was to live with Dad. She probably came to that conclusion as my sister tried helping Dad with Mom as things progressively got worse. Mom viewed her as having ulterior motives and a threat. It is hard for the family to accept these type of accusations, even when you know there is no basis for them.

Life for Dad with Mom grew more and more strenuous each day with continuous accusations and paranoia taking over. Neither Mom or Dad slept well. Their day was spent watching TV and Dad trying to figure out how and what they would eat. When the memory care facility called with an open room that summer, Dad initially said it wasn't time, but then reality set in and he reluctantly agreed. It was the hardest thing he ever had to do. The guilt he felt in not being able to care for his wife was what kept him from seeking help before now. My conversation with Dad was one of assurance that he was doing what he needed to do for his own health. I firmly stated that he was still her caregiver and would still make decisions for Mom, but that the facility would do the hard work.

His job now was to be able to spend time with Mom without arguments. He no longer had to fight her to bathe or get her dressed appropriately. He no longer had to figure out what to do for dinner or how to run errands with her by his side. He no longer would have her following him every step with suspicion.

Getting Help

Devotion:

Why do we believe we can do things on our own? Pride becomes a stumbling block in seeing the truth. Society tells us that we can and should do it all. The world told Dad a good husband would take care of her. He believed in his solemn oath, his sacred vow, to take care of her in good times and bad, to take care of her in sickness and health.

Would giving in be breaking the vow to his wife? Was he giving up on her? We can do all thing through Christ who strengthens us. (Philippians 4:13) Pride refers to self and self-exultation. What Dad felt was not pride at all. He completely gave of himself to do everything possible to help his wife. It took humility to admit he could no longer do so. And in doing so, he did not give up on her but gave both her and himself new life. She had started a new life. She is taken care of, shown love, allowed to laugh and interact with others. He was able to begin taking care of himself. Now when he goes to visit, they can enjoy themselves without worrying about all the necessities. God provides. Sometimes we need to step away so we can see what God is doing in our lives and what is the next step to follow.

Chapter 9

A New Way of Life

Summer, 2015

Dad cried just about all the time. He is mourning, his heart broken. He had lost his wife, but she was not dead. Reality began to set in. No more would she accompany him to church, go on vacations with him, or have a regular, ordinary conversation. Those days were over. It was hard for him to go out of the house without her, to go to church or the store. His life had forever changed. His college aged grandson was able to stay with him for a month after Mom moved out. This was a great relief to have some activity in this now quiet house.

Although she didn't recognize the place she now lived in as a "facility," she did at first ask to go home. We needed to remind Dad that she asked to go home even when she was home. Thankfully, this didn't last long. We tried putting pictures of her family all around, but it didn't really seem to faze her. She didn't even glance at the photos to see if she recognized anyone. She doesn't feel at home anywhere, anymore. We have all adjusted to this new kind of life. Several times a day, she is lead to her room, where she knocks on the door and peaks in. She has to

A New Way of Life

be reassured it is OK to go into the room. She is hesitant to go in or sit on the furniture. The same is true when she visits her home periodically. She is lead around the house, and she peaks through all the doors looking for the bathroom. Nothing is familiar to her. Can you imagine being in a constant state of confusion, not knowing where you are, who to trust, or where you should lay your head at night?

I often wonder what she thinks of while she is there, if she has any thoughts at all. She lives in the moment and can participate somewhat in activities. It was still apparent to family and caregivers whether she did or did not like something. Her emotions and reactions were still intact. Part of her was still with us and we thanked God for the part of her that we still held on to.

Dad finds some relief through an Alzheimer's Support Group. It only meets once a month, and he wishes they could meet more. It is here that he hears from experts on this disease and learns how many others have been or are currently going through the same thing. He recognizes where he has been and wants to know more. It is a safe place for people to express what they are wrestling with in this disease and where others understand.

Early on in the facility, if she were asked what she had been doing all day, she would go through a list of how she had gone to work, getting a lot of things done, then had been running errands.

Mom loves music, and it has been an outlet for her. Music and dancing somehow keeps Mom and Dad connected, even when they can't communicate. As long as she will be physically able, Dad will dance with her. When there seems to be nothing, she comes alive when music is played. She mostly responds to church hymns, patriotic songs, and Elvis. Her eyes glaze over more and more. Not usually when there is music. Suddenly she can sing and dance. What a thrill it is to Dad to still have this part of her with him.

An Introspective Journey

One of Mom's favorite activities was coloring. She felt productive, often acting as if she were working on a project. Her desire to be purposeful and productive was still being lived out. Often she walked around the facility, picking up a pen and paper and just write. She no longer can put ideas or words together in writing, but she would trace or copy words already on a page. She held herself with such dignity as if she fully knew what she was doing. She often wrote her name or that of a loved one. It was the one thing she could still do, something she remembered. When she noticed the sign in sheet at the front desk, she would sign her name or that of a family member.

She talked less. She had trouble following a conversation, so when she talked, it didn't always flow. There were times, out of nowhere, she started talking as if she were in the middle of a conversation that wasn't happening. She no longer asks to go home or realizes she is in another place. I'm not sure how I feel about that.

Chapter 10

Never Give Up

Summer, 2016

One morning Dad received a call from the facility concerned about the lack of responsiveness Mom was having. They needed to help her walk, and her mouth was drooling. Something was not right. We all feared a stroke. We rushed over and drove her to the emergency room. I've never seen a group of people work so quickly in diagnosing the problem. After a few brief tests, they concluded she had indeed had a stroke. She was also dehydrated. Once the IV had given her strength back, she was ready to get up and leave. The doctors were prepared to let her go after she could successfully drink some fluids. It was discovered at this time, she couldn't swallow. They kept her overnight. It was determined she could return to her facility but would need drinks thickened and her food pureed. She could no longer talk. How confused she must have been.

Months later with therapy, she was able to move to chopped foods and thickened liquids. Her language has come back to a small extent, but will never be able to hold a conversation again. She can say words or phrases at times. She's a bit slower moving around and no longer colors. She needs assistance in all aspects of grooming. She is shown where to go and what to do. She rarely spontaneously joins in with others without assistance although she is drawn to a crowd and will walk over to see what is going on. She has that "on the go" instinct. She will be in a group and just decide to get up and walk around. She is curious and is attracted to crowds, music, and activities. She also still loves beautiful things. One day, Dad walked into her room to find a beautiful vase of flowers. He asked the nurse who had sent the flowers. She went to the room to check it out. She laughed as she told Dad those flowers had been on her desk. Mom liked them so much; she brought them to her room. She still appreciates beauty.

Mom is still compassionate. She goes to the patients in the facility that are in wheelchairs and pushes them around. (Whether they want her to or not.) When she is in one of the classes they offer, Mom will straighten up the papers and tries to tend to the others in need. She might not know where she is or what she is doing, but she is still there in her own way. One Monday one of the workers came in with a gift for Mom, a baby stroller she had found at a garage sale. Mom pushes the stroller all around the facility. It gives her purpose, thinking she is helping in some way. Of course, she also leaves it in different places around the facility, but they just kindly return it to her room. She can't do what she used to, but we rejoice in seeing her sweet spirit in the things she does do.

Mom is now disconnected from her family. The family gatherings still happen. Sometimes we bring her where we are, or we go to her. She no longer knows who we are and doesn't engage in the event. She is missing out on the joy of her family. In a way she is in one world and we are all in another. But there are still times without warning, she responds to something. This past summer, out of the blue, she looked at me and slowly, laboriously said "my daughter, Paula." Tears welled in my eyes. She knew me, she called me by name. Then in a flash, the recognition was gone. Sometimes she will laugh at the right time, or to join in an activity. Recently, we were walking around in the memory care facility, and she noticed the group hitting a balloon to each other in a circle. She turned and asked as clear as possible, "Why are they doing that?" I answered, "I suppose it is because they are having fun. Do you want to join them?" She shook her head yes and followed directions to participate for a short while.

This is not the life they planned Mom and Dad had as they grew old together. However, it is what it is. We celebrate the small things; the smile she might show or simply letting Dad hold her hand or join him in a dance. This disease doesn't diminish the love they shared or the life they lived together. It is a long good-bye. She is here and at the same time she isn't. I miss my mom. I miss having long conversations with her, asking for her advice, getting her point of view on issues, and sharing victories in our lives. We have lost a wife, a mother, and a friend, but she is happy. She is kind and compassionate with others around her. We believe she is at peace. Her life has been unforgettable. We will hold her example of how to live and how to love others selflessly. Her surrender to let her life be as God planned it, never giving up and giving God the Glory.

Devotion

I think about this disease and what it does to each person and the families affected by Alzheimer's. Many of us wonder what hope looks like. There is comfort in the Word of God.

An Introspective Journey

2 Corinthians 4:16
> "We do not lose heart. Though outwardly we are wasting away, yet inwardly we are being renewed day by day."

I rather like the way Eugene Peterson paraphrases this scripture in The Message, "We're not giving up. How could we! Even though on the outside it often looks like things are falling apart on us, on the inside, where God is making new life, not a day goes by without his unfolding grace."

Grace is always stronger than our circumstances. It becomes comforting to me in knowing that although outwardly, she appears to have lost it all, inwardly, Christ is renewing her. I must believe, just because she can't express herself, it doesn't mean God isn't alive and well in her soul. The pain we feel inside from this disease is real, but it does not negate the joy the Lord offers and promises. Joy is also real. Mom knew this disease was ravishing her mind but still embraced her faith as she voluntarily expressed her devotion to God by accepting this. I am comforted in knowing Mom is not in any pain; she seems to be at peace. We hold on to the moments we have with her. They are becoming fewer and fewer. We know there all we have. But we refuse to give up on her.

There is still a powerful joy that lives inside of her that nothing can take away. It's a sacred, secret laughter that creeps out of her without any prompting. She may be sitting or standing, in a crowd or by herself. She will just start to laugh. She can't talk and doesn't really responding to anyone or anything, but that laughter, that joy from inside of her just emerges with the best smile she can make out. This laughter brings a tear to my eyes and I know I've gotten a glimpse of Christ's joy that is still alive inside of this body that many have written off. This joy, this peace that surrounds our souls can bring healing to our troubles and sorrows.

Once she told me she was thankful her mother had Alzheimer's. She described her mother's life as sad and unhappy. With Alzheimer's her mother no longer lived in turmoil, but had this time of peace before she died. God is always good, especially when we don't understand. It is Christ who gives us the strength and courage to hang on when we want to quit. Christ gives us peace and hope through our struggle. God doesn't will for anyone to suffer through diseases such as Alzheimer's. His will is for our good. Even when life plays a dirty trick on us riddling with disease and evil, our God reigns and carries us through.

As Mom's decline became more apparent, I missed her more every day. I missed our deep conversations—I missed her laughter, her wisdom, her joy. I longed for another moment with her, just one more special time between the two of us. It had been so long since we connected. I asked God to grant me a selfish wish, to have another moment with Mom. We've all heard stories of someone near death waking up, becoming lucid, and speaking to a loved one briefly. I believed with all my heart, if it were in His will, God would grant me my request. So I waited for this moment, wondering if she would suddenly say a word, look at me and smile, or even better, I wondered if it were to come in a dream where we would walk around together having a last intimate conversation as we'd done in the past.

Shortly after this prayer, I had the opportunity to spend the day with Mom in the memory care unit. I fed her, talked to her, and walked her around. Watching her struggle with simple things reminded me so much of a little child who needs help and encouragement to do the most basic tasks. Her empty eyes wandered as I tried to capture a glimmer of her soul trapped inside her body. I was looking for that moment I'd asked for.

She started responding some during music activities for the residents that day. It was near July 4th, and common areas were decorated with stars and stripes with red, white, and blue around every corner. The room filled with patriotic music being sung with enthusiasm by their music teacher. Mom was responding to the music, tapping her foot and was trying to clap with help. At this point, even responding to music is fading and short lived.

I basked being in her presence as she was mildly engaged. She sat in a comfortable chair, and I sat on the floor by her feet encouraging her participation. I held her hand when our eyes met as she looked down at me with an overwhelming flow of love. I froze, taking in every moment. She took her hand and gently cupped it around my face as she continued looking into my eyes. She couldn't talk, but she didn't need to. Her eyes talked for her. I felt her love,;I felt the love of Christ flowing from her. I didn't see anger, frustration, pain, or fear. I somehow knew, she was no longer struggling, but was at peace and wanted me to be at peace also. Not wanting the moment to end, I soaked up the love she was showing me.

The following week I found these words in one of Mom's journals in response to I John 4:11-18:

1 John 4:11-18 (NIV)

> Dear friends, since God so loved us, we also ought to love one another. No one has ever seen God; but if we love one another, God lives in us and his love is made complete in us. This is how we know that we live in him and he in us: He has given us of his Spirit. And we have seen and testify that the Father

has sent his Son to be the Savior of the world. If anyone acknowledges that Jesus is the Son of God, God lives in them and they in God. And so we know and rely on the love God has for us. God is love. Whoever lives in love lives in God, and God in them. This is how love is made complete among us so that we will have confidence on the day of judgment: In this world we are like Jesus. There is no fear in love. But perfect love drives out fear because fear has to do with punishment. The one who fears is not made perfect in love.

"When we love one another, we love God. God loves through the people and circumstances and events in our lives. His love comes into perfection in us. Receiving and giving little kindnesses even the mere presence of another is loving; like couples growing so familiar with each other that there is no need for words."

This gift of grace from Christ was more than I asked for, more than I imagined. I think, "It doesn't get any better than this! I just experienced the extravagant love Christ offers us here on Earth." At that moment, there were 3 of us there. Me, Mom, and the presence of the Holy Spirit. Mom's earthly connection with us now is minimal, but I believe her relationship, her connection with Christ, is limitless. Perhaps she spends time dancing and singing in heaven while her unresponsive body is still here. No, Mom doesn't act the same or look the same as when this disease did not afflict her. But, yes, she is there. The spirit of love that made her who she was, still dwells within her. That is something this disease can never take away.

God prepared her for this journey years before it took over who she was, and He has never left her. She prayed to God that

An Introspective Journey

if she were to live with this disease, that she could help others through her suffering. That is the reason for this publication. Know you are not alone, seek help from others, and enjoy life in the big and little things. We have a choice on how to respond when life happens. I choose to thank God for the time we have had with Mom. I choose to seek joy in every situation, and I choose to find small blessings every day. Bitterness will only break my spirit and bring torment me. My prayer is for others not to have to go through this. But if you must face this, ask Christ to be your counselor and guide, your Prince of Peace. We have learned that through it all his eyes are on us and all will be well.

One day she will cross that bridge from life to death to new life. It is there that she will finally have that sense of "homecoming." She will feel welcomed and have that "at-home" feeling, that feeling that all is right and familiar. She will relax and be at peace with her Savior.

Facts about Alzheimer's Disease

FROM THE ALZHEIMER'S ASSOCIATION

An estimated 5.7 million people are living with Alzheimer's Disease in 2018. Every 65 seconds someone in the United states develops the disease. It is the 6th leading cause of death in the United States. It is also the only top 10 cause of death in the US that cannot be prevented, cured, or even slowed. 1 in 3 seniors die with Alzheimer's or other forms of dementia. There are more deaths from Alzheimer's Disease than breast cancer and prostate cancer together.

Alzheimer's Association:
https://www.alz.org/alzheimers-dementia/facts-figures

About the Author

Paula Sarver believes that life is a journey meant to be shared and lived in the richness of kindness, compassion, and joy that only comes from above.

Her passion is serving Christ and spreading the news of how much each of us is unconditionally loved by our Father in heaven. She knows in the most difficult times, Christ has never failed or abandoned her. She desires others to know that same hope and comfort that is available for all.

She has a Master's degree in education and has worked in the public school system for more than a quarter-century. Her focus is on helping struggling students, building their capacity to become successful adults reaching their potential.

Paula was born in Texas, grew up in South Louisiana, and now calls Tennessee home. She resides in Knoxville with her loving husband, Daniel. They have two adult boys, Stephen and Jacob.

Also Available From

WordCrafts Press

Geezer Stories: *The Care & Feeding of Old People*
   Laura Mansfield

Against Every Hope: *India, Mother Teresa, and a Baby Girl*
   Bonnie Tinsley

Embracing a New Vision of Aging
   Sheryl Towers

Elders at the Gate: *A Call to Repair the Generational Links*
   Ray Blunt

www.wordcrafts.net

www.ingramcontent.com/pod-product-compliance
Lightning Source LLC
Chambersburg PA
CBHW052133110526
44591CB00012B/1707